YOGA

FOR THE

INFLEXIBLE

MALE

YOGA MATT

YOGA
FOR THE
INFLEXIBLE
MALE

A HOW-TO GUIDE

illustrations by Richard Sheppard

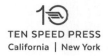

TEN SPEED PRESS
California | New York

Contents

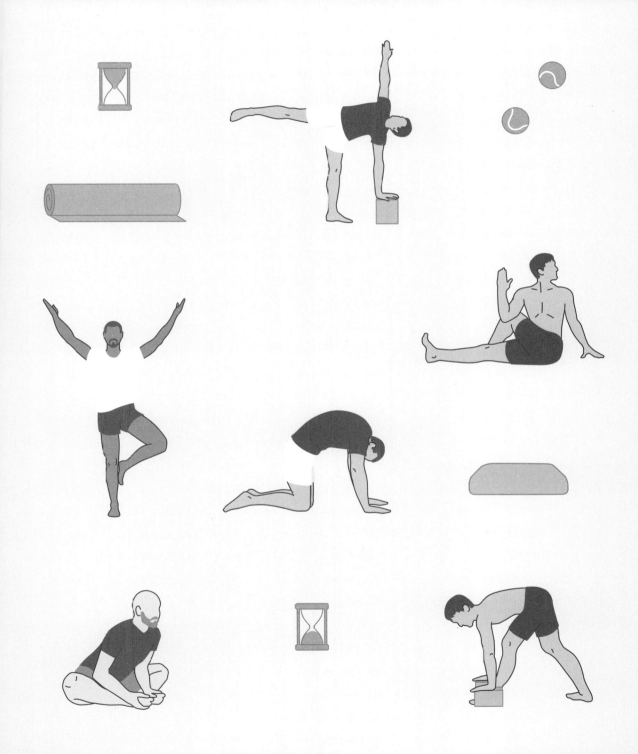

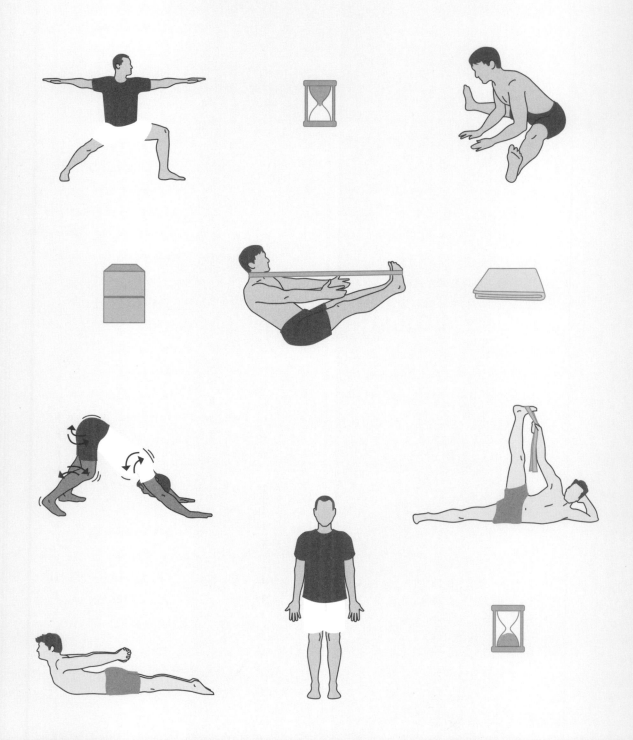

Foreword

I knew Yoga Matt before he was Yoga Matt. He was just Roy, a humorous guy with a great idea—a yoga class designed for men.

I began studying yoga more than twenty years ago, and every class I've ever taken or taught has been attended by more women than men. Luring men into the studio has always been a challenge, and this means that half the population is missing out on all the benefits—physical, mental, and emotional—that a yoga practice brings. I knew Roy's idea for a men's-only class would fill a void.

Luckily, we already had the perfect teacher for the class at our studio—Jerry Sinclair. From his own experience as an athlete, a yoga practitioner, and an instructor, Jerry knows how to modify traditional poses for the most inflexible among us, which makes yoga accessible to everyone, including men.

The approach to yoga in this book is funny and friendly, but don't be fooled by the light tone. All the instructions are accurate and detailed. Yoga Matt, or Roy, or whatever he calls himself, is not just a comedian; he's also a good writer. That, combined with Jerry's genius pose modifications, makes this the perfect book for a man—or anyone—who wants to try yoga but hasn't felt confident enough to step into a studio.

I hope *Yoga for the Inflexible Male* is the beginning of a lifelong yoga practice for you that is full of flexibility, joy, laughter, peace, and growth.

—**Jenn Russo**
  Co-owner of Yoga on Center
  Healdsburg and Cloverdale, California

A Few Words from Yoga Matt

A funny thing happened when the new yoga studio, Yoga on Center, came to town. Mainly, that I started doing yoga. You'd think somebody named Yoga would be more familiar with the ancient art, but, hey, it's only a family name. I'm as inflexible as the rest of us. This is the story of how an inflexible male became a lot more flexible, and it could become your story, too.

The thought of practicing yoga had dimly crossed my radar. I'm athletic, a compulsive bike rider. Yet for all the miles I log in the saddle, I wouldn't call myself *limber*. I'd require an ambulance standing by in order to perform the feat of bending over to touch my toes. The idea of flexibility appealed, but the mental image of practicing yoga in front of women did not. I'm sorry: I have my pride. The class I envisioned would be men only. A kind of bring me your stiff, your deeply embarrassed, your previously yoga-phobic.

Yoga on Center surprisingly agreed. Then something else surprising happened. The class immediately sold out. A second class was added, also selling out. Same story in their other studios. Apparently, there is a fairly large but latent section of the male population interested in the ancient practice—if the class was solely for inflexible men.

Now every Tuesday and Friday at four p.m. a brave contingent of men put on their yoga pants and file into Yoga on Center. Well, to be honest, nobody wears yoga pants in this crowd. Shorts and T-shirts are the rule. It's a room full of men who look like they might be going to the market for a half gallon of milk. Rookies, one and all, blissfully ignorant of the term *downward dog*, which very well might refer to a depressed canine in need of mood enhancers. Injuries abound. Trick knees, wonky backs, a panoply of sports-related boo-boos. The bodies might not be entirely willing, but the overall spirit is.

Jerry is our fearless teacher, an athletic seventy-year-old with a bushy mustache and the avuncular bearing of a wrestling coach. A number of years ago, doctors informed him he'd need to walk with a cane for the rest of his life. Jerry chose yoga instead. Not only does he walk perfectly well, but he's also capable of bending himself into some insanely freaky positions.

For our class, Jerry is gentle and encouraging in his instruction. He demonstrates a pose, and the class, to varying degrees of pliancy, imitates his example. Jerry thankfully keeps his corrections to a minimum. The goal isn't to strike the perfect pose, but to embrace the *wabi sabi*–ness of it all. Inhibitions gradually recede. Muscles are stretched and prodded. The rest of the world goes away. We can't pronounce the names of the poses, but we're doing them, and a palpable spirit of *hey, look ma, no hands* permeates the air. For a bunch of unyielding middle-aged men, it's quite remarkable.

This book captures that experience, Jerry included. It's not meant to be an encyclopedic tome about yoga. If I can speak on behalf of those with XY chromosomes, we don't care about that stuff. *Yoga for the Inflexible Male* is intended to give you what you need to improve your flexibility, with plenty of pictures, because as everyone knows, guys like pictures.

The chapters are divided into three hourlong practices, each comprised of twelve to seventeen poses. One pose transitions into the next. A handy graphic illustrates the good way to do the pose, the not-so-bad, and the ugly—the no-frills, basic down-and-dirty. In the back of the book, there's a section for combining poses from different sessions for sport-specific practices.

Yoga for the Inflexible Male is designed to lie flat for easy reference while you're on the yoga mat. Maybe practice in front of a mirror to ensure you're doing it right. You'll soon discover yoga isn't so different from weight training, except your body's the weight and you're working more on balance, not bulking up. Added bonus: It's also more peaceful than a weight room and requires way less equipment. All you need is this book, a body, a yoga mat, and a willingness to try something new. You'll still be a guy, but with yoga, you'll be a lot less inflexible of body. And perhaps of spirit, too. That's what happened to me.

One more thing. I'm just the microphone here. I'll be the first to admit it: I'm no expert. Just a goofy guy who came up with the idea for the class. The rest is all Jerry and he has credentials up the wazoo.

Don't let that crazy mustache fool you. He brings decades of wisdom to our world of beginner male yoga every week. I've tape recorded each class. I know, probably illegal in a few states. But it was the only way I could capture every nuance of Jerry's expertise.

All the jokes—good and bad—are mine. Jerry's funny, but not intentionally. I mean no harm. My aim is to entertain and include everyone. It's not truly funny unless everyone's laughing. Often I'm just poking fun at myself, the prototypical inflexible male. The rest is pure joy for yoga. Out of shyness and male bashfulness about looking inept, I thought life was going to pass me by without experiencing the ancient practice. Happily, that didn't happen.

I'm a modest practitioner of the trade, but if I'm any indication of what yoga can do, here's the kind of hard data that men appreciate. My average on the bike is a mile per hour faster. Hills and wind are smaller obstacles and I regularly outride cyclists twenty years my junior, laughing to myself as I pass them. It's all natural, none of those performance enhancers. When other riders ask me what my secret is, all I tell them is it's a four-letter word.

PROPS

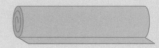

YOGA MAT

A bit of basic training is in order before you get started. A number of props are used in yoga, and it's helpful to know what their purpose is and how to employ them. It's also helpful to know that yoga can be done without these props—and that many household items can be used instead in a pinch.

Starting from the ground up, let's consider the **yoga mat**. Jerry likes to call it a "sticky mat," which is more descriptive (although I think yoga mat is a perfectly good name). It's a reference to the rubber surface that provides adhesion, so you don't slip while performing poses.

Compared to wrestling or tumbling mats, yoga mats are spartan in terms of padding, but that's the idea. You aren't going to be performing flips. Most of the poses, in fact, are stationary, and the thinness of the surface allows your body to maintain optimal balance. Yoga can be done without a mat, but mats provide cushioning and some traction when balancing in poses.

Another handy piece of equipment is the **yoga block**. Jerry says that when he was starting out—in the horse-and-buggy age of yoga—the blocks were made of wood. Nowadays, they're made of a lighter composite material. It's mentioned a couple of times in this book that you could simply substitute

YOGA BLOCK

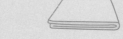

YOGA BLANKET

YOGA BOLSTER

YOGA STRAP

a thick hardback book for the same purpose, binding the covers together with tape. But if you might want to read the book someday, a yoga block is handier. Blocks are great because they can give you height and lever-age, especially if you're on the inflexible side.

The **yoga blanket** is thick and has a dense weave and is probably too rough for sleep-ing. If you're kneeling on the mat, however, your knees will thank you when you cush-ion them with a blanket. A beach towel is a fine substitute.

The **yoga bolster** is a tool for providing a helpful modification to traditional yoga poses; it's basically an extra-firm pillow. Sitting cross-legged on a bolster allows your hips to be higher than your knees, the correct orienta-tion. It's also thicker and denser than a normal couch bolster, and the person you live with might prefer to keep that piece of upholstery on the sofa.

A **yoga strap** is an essential tool in class. It extends the reach of your arm, for example, in those poses where you're down on the mat and reaching to grab a toe at the end of an extended leg. Unless you own some Jerry-like flexibility, a strap—a length of ribbed nylon belted with a plastic cinch at one end—is a godsend. A fabric belt or rubber resistance band can be a good substitute here.

The yoga studio has a collection of all of these. The typical setup in class is a mat, two blocks, three blankets, a bolster, and a strap. For home use, that might sound like a lot, but it's actually less expensive than most well-used bicycles you could buy on the internet. In the long run, it amounts to a small investment for a practice that can improve your life for as long as you live. And you can also use what you already have and then buy props over time to spread out the cost.

MORE PROPS TO YOU

These props are not made for yoga specifically but are still helpful.

TIMER

Jerry uses one so he doesn't fall asleep during *savasana*.

TENNIS BALLS

A great massager. Sit on them and roll around. Ahh. Now in the small of your back, then higher.

DOWEL

Sawn from common wooden dowels found at hardware stores. Offers killer foot massage. Always pick up after use to avoid a slip-on-banana-peel situation.

How to Use This Book

| 0 to 20 Minutes | 21 to 40 Minutes | 41 to 60 Minutes |

Use this somewhat obsolete device as a reminder not to rush through each practice. They're divided into roughly 20-minute segments for you to recalibrate to maintain a slow and steady path. When the sand runs out, you're done. (You'll be deep in *savasana* by then. What's *savasana*? See the glossary.)

Each Manly Practice runs about an hour. There's no such thing as speed yoga. The mantra throughout is slow and steady. Ideally, two times a week is a good frequency, so your muscles don't have time to forget what they just learned.

To keep you from blasting through each practice, we've included an hourglass icon at roughly 20-minute intervals throughout the practice for you to calibrate your inner clock and serve as a reminder to slow down on the mat. It's all about reminding you to breathe. There's an old saying in yoga: breath follows motion. In practice that means inhaling gives you the energy to twist yourself into some really impressive shapes, while exhaling immediately relaxes you from that exertion. It's the perfect partnership. In other words, every pose begins and ends with breathing, like a circle.

In addition to the running hourglass figure, at the front of each practice there's a graphic for the props you'll need for the next hour. That way you don't have to get up from your mat to fetch them and break your concentration. You're welcome. Also, the book binding has been designed for opening flat right in front of you for handy reference.

Jerry has a little formula for the order of his *asanas* (poses). It's a closely held secret, so don't tell anybody who hasn't bought this book. He begins the class with a focus on the breath, which segues into several gentle warm-up poses, and then the real yoga begins. The poses get more vigorous, and then eventually step back to a warming-down phase, which is different from cooling down. The muscles continue to be engaged rather than in a state of rest. Around this time Jerry usually introduces a twist. Then last, it's *savasana* time, the cherry on top of your yoga practice—a period of restorative rest that leaves you in perfect physical and mental alignment for reentering the world outside your room.

Some of the Manly Practices have more poses than others. That's just because some *asanas*, such as mountain pose, are great jumping-off points for a number of different poses.

You'll also notice that each Manly Practice features a different version of downward dog. We're not stinting you here. Yoga Matt would never do that. These dogs are quite different from one another in terms of how you perform them and the props used. The other thing, *dawg*, is that downward dog is aimed at two particularly manly trouble spots: hamstrings and shoulders. Our legs have to carry us around all day and our shoulders are where we store stress.

The Sanskrit name—unless it's a pose of Jerry's own invention—is almost always included. It's a matter of respect. I don't want to cue the New Age music or anything, but yoga's an ancient art and using the actual word takes you back to its venerable roots. Back in those days, they didn't use mats or bolsters or straps. Those guys were old school. They just used their bodies.

Most of the words, like *asana*, end with an *a*. If you're like ol' Yoga Matt, *savasana* will be the first one that sticks in the brainpan because it just involves lying back on your mat and breathing. Most *asanas* come with three versions, the good, the not-so-bad, and the ugly. The ugly really isn't ugly. You're getting the same benefits without straining. The truth is, if you regularly practice yoga, it's all good no matter how limber you are.

The steady motto of this book is *no pain, no pain*. Resist doing the regular guy thing and going in the red zone. That's not yoga. That's stupid. You don't want to invite injury. Yoga isn't a sport. It's more rightly called a practice because it's not just a body thing. The mind is engaged and quieted, working in unison with your body, which is a rare occurrence for most of us. Remember, breath follows motion. Your body will do the rest.

History of Yoga

Yoga goes back a long, long way. Even before someone decided it was probably a good idea to wear helmets when playing tackle football. You have to turn your time machine back to the year 3000 BCE. So, give or take, the ancient practice is like five thousand years old.

It all started in India. The specifics are kind of hazy, but it was probably a bunch of guys standing around, thinking a health club might be a good idea. One without any specialized equipment, of course, because that wasn't invented yet. So they developed a simple, elegant method for exercising the body and mind. Around 400 BCE, someone named Patanjali decided to write it all down, which formed the origins of the poses in this book.

Like any good idea, it spread across boundaries, religions, and cultures, developing into a variety of yoga schools. There's Hatha yoga, with a focus on steady pace and balance. Ashtanga yoga is quick-paced. Iyengar yoga is for precision and alignment. In Vinyasa yoga, one pose flows into another. In other words, a whole bunch of different ways to get bent. There's even something called goat yoga! Don't worry. We don't practice any of that here. This book is rated strictly NG (no goat).

Even though yoga's been part of Hindu and Buddhist belief for millennia, it didn't really become a religion in the United States until fairly recently. In the 1970s, the early adopters were often associated with granola and broken-down VW buses—a period referred to by many as the "dark ages" of yoga.

Then in the 1990s, yoga became a fixture in our culture, first primarily with women. Men, meanwhile, remained ignorant of the ancient practice until yoga began to infiltrate training routines of professional athletes. Still, as a tribe, we were scared. What if I look stupid? Aren't women better at it than me? Will I have to grow a beard?

Thankfully, Jerry's more evolved than most men. He saw the light early on about yoga, almost thirty years ago. He's a manly man—surfer, wrestler, builder—and has a lot of manly injuries as a result. Jerry eventually branched out into studying a variety of schools of yoga, and he brings that breadth of knowledge to this book. There are traditional Hatha poses that date back five thousand years. Some poses are pure Vinyasa yoga, flowing from one *asana* to another like the freaking Ganges River. Plus other moves you won't find anywhere else, developed by Jerry to address his own assortment of accumulated sports injuries. Each one is a manly pose that will make you more, well, manly.

MANLY YOGA PRACTICE NO. 1

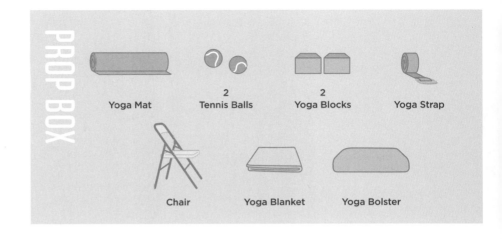

PROP BOX

Yoga Mat

2 Tennis Balls

2 Yoga Blocks

Yoga Strap

Chair

Yoga Blanket

Yoga Bolster

Your first series of poses—*asanas*—are totally hip. By that I mean, that's what they loosen and stretch. Your hips, not to mention your hamstrings. Each movement within this series flows gently to the next, so right off the bat, you're doing what's called Vinyasa yoga. Pretty impressive. Feel free to throw these terms around in mixed company.

Have a couple of tennis balls handy, because the practice starts off with a Jerry special. A strap should be handy, too. A couple of yoga blocks (or thick books that you'll never read) will be put to good use. Now, ol' Yoga Matt's assuming you already have a yoga mat. A blanket or two folded in half on top of the mat is good for people with knee issues.

Always take your time. Don't go all Usain Bolt. Slow and steady wins the yoga race. This should take an hour, but don't be a clock-watcher. Follow your breath. It will lead you where you need to go.

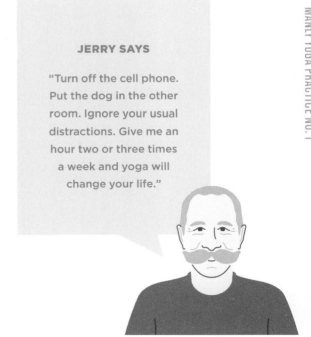

JERRY SAYS

"Turn off the cell phone. Put the dog in the other room. Ignore your usual distractions. Give me an hour two or three times a week and yoga will change your life."

Balls and Straps

Resist the dopey ball joke. This is a great opening stretch. Anyone can do it—and it's good however you do it. Jerry brings the tennis balls to class in a box that's been sitting in the sun: nice and warm for where they're going.

Lie on your back, knees bent, feet on the floor. Now is a good time to begin the calm, easy breath that will carry you through the practice. Take the two tennis balls and place one on each side of your tailbone, a hand's width apart. Roll around on top of them, concentrating on areas that feel tight. Really work out the knots. Then slide down on your mat so the balls are midback, finding spots that "need attention," as Jerry says. If you feel like it, scoot down further so the balls are at your shoulder blades. (The no-ball joke still applies.) Try placing them at the base of the skull. You might need to hold 'em there with your fingers.

Last, place the balls under your buns. (You know what I mean.) Grab a yoga strap (or the belt from when you were the fat you). Your left leg remains straight on the floor. Your right knee bends toward your chest. With your right hand on your knee, rotate the knee around. Slow big circles; clockwise, then counterclockwise. Remove balls when done.

JERRY SAYS

"When I say core, I mean those deep belly muscles. You know, the ones under your six-pack."

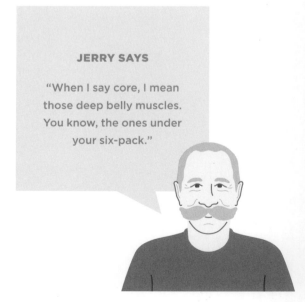

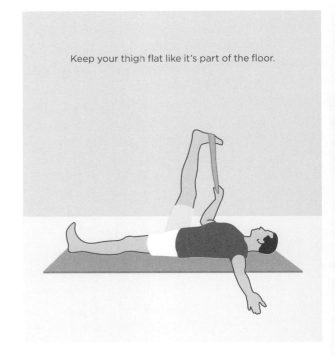

Keep your thigh flat like it's part of the floor.

Next, place the yoga strap around the sole of your right foot. Extend your right leg up like a straight knife blade. Bring it as high as you can above your body, each hand grasping an end of the strap, arms straight, legs straight. Hold the pose while you take a few slow and steady yoga breaths. Then put both ends of the strap in your right hand. Extend your left arm out to the side, like you're pointing at something over there. With balls nestled under buns this whole time, take your right leg to the right without the left thigh coming off the floor. Jerry often suggests you imagine an elephant on your thigh. He has a thing about elephants. But what he means is, keep that thigh down! If you can't, then keep your right leg up higher.

To come out of the pose, use your core—your abs—to swivel the right leg back over your body. Keep the ends of the strap in your right hand. We're not done yet. Take your right leg across your body to your left.

Don't go so far that your hip rises from the floor. Hold the position for a few breaths. Use your core again to pull yourself out of the move. Remove the strap. Lower your right leg on the floor.

Oh yeah. Now do all that with the left leg. Elephant on right thigh this time. Both legs, according to Jerry, should feel the same when done.

Seated Salute Pose and Hero Pose (*Virasana*) with Forward Bend

The next four poses are all similar. Each is a very *hip* hip opener. They're also good for your hamstrings, each stretching your muscles in a different way.

Hero pose—or *virasana*—is guaranteed to put more flexibility in your hips, hammies, and knees, too. If you have knee issues, do this entire sequence sitting cross-legged on a bolster. Also have two yoga blocks—or thick hardcover books—within reach.

Start the pose on your hands and knees, with a blanket under your knees, if needed. Keep your knees together like a hinge and separate your feet wide enough to fit a block between your ankles. Sit back on the block. Lift the skin of your knees, move your calves out of the way, and ground your shins, giving you a solid base to work from.

Next, to borrow a refrain from your mother, sit up straight. Position your elbows at your sides, palms resting on your thighs, and open your chest. Separate your sit bones. Wait, what? "It's more of a muscular thing," Jerry explains. "Pull the left side to the left, the right to the right."

Keep your head evenly balanced over your collarbones and chin level, then lengthen the spine by pulling your abs in. Lift your trunk—the sides, not the ribs—upward while relaxing the tailbone down. At the same time, unclench your shoulders and let them drop. The crown of the head reaches for the ceiling. Soften your spine and allow it to move into your body (again, a muscular movement, not surgery). You should be just sitting, breathing, quieting the mind. Cool air in, slightly warmer air out. Put the palms of your hands together, fingers spread, thumbs to chest. Don't collapse your chest. Lift it, then drop your chin to meet it. Jerry always says the word *namaskarasana* at this point. "It's not prayer pose," he admonishes, "it's salute pose." Don't ask. It kind of ruins the moment. Just do what Jerry says.

Then grab the unused block (the one you're not sitting on). Make sure you're maintaining that make-your-mother-proud posture. Squeeze the block between your hands. Hold your hands with the block out in front of you, sleepwalker style. Now rotate your arms up to twelve o'clock. Your biceps should be all the way back by your ears. Keep your arms straight and your shoulders down. Don't forget to continue to squeeze the block or it'll drop on your head.

For the grand finale, bring your arms back down. You can put the block aside. Starting with hands at your sides, walk them forward on the mat in front of you. Jerry reminds us at this point to breathe into the front and back of the lungs. Another one of his metaphors; I don't actually think that's anatomically possible.

On the exhale, walk your hands further out until you find a bit of resistance, then stop and inhale into it to soften the resistance. Don't go any further. "If the tightness goes away," Jerry says, "enjoy it." Then slowly walk your hands back to your thighs as you sit up. No sudden movements. It's yoga, not the hundred-yard dash.

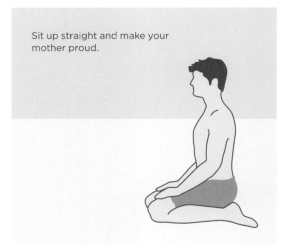

Sit up straight and make your mother proud.

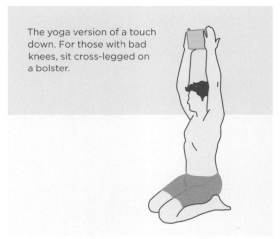

The yoga version of a touch down. For those with bad knees, sit cross-legged on a bolster.

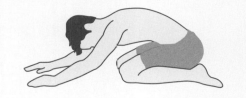

For those with an inner Gumby, go for it. If your breathing is labored, walk the hands back. You've gone too far.

Staff Pose (*Dandasana*) with Forward Bend (*Paschimottanasana*)

Dandasana, **or staff pose, is the second in our series of four symmetrical poses that are particularly good for loosening the hips.** Sit on the floor, legs out in front of you. Most guys, because they have tight hamstrings, will prefer to sit on a blanket or two, a block, or a bolster. Whatever you need to get your pelvis straight up and your legs straight out. Position yourself on the edge of your perch, legs out in front of you, feet pointing up, big toes touching.

Push your feet away from you without pointing or curling your toes. Try to reach with your heels. Engage the muscles around your shins and thigh bones, pull your kneecaps back toward your waist, and pull the backs of your knees toward the floor. Lengthen your spine and reach with the crown of your head for the ceiling. As before, take a block (or an extra copy of *Ulysses*), squeeze it between your hands, and hold it out in front of you, arms straight and outstretched for a moment. Raise the block above your head, keeping your arms straight, until your arms are next to your ears.

At this point in the pose, Jerry suggests, "See if you can breathe." Of course, you can. He means that steady and calm yoga breath. No panting. (This isn't downward dog.) Then slowly bring your arms back down in front of you and deposit the block/book on the floor, still keeping your posture.

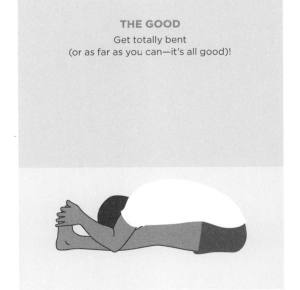

THE GOOD
Get totally bent
(or as far as you can—it's all good)!

The next part is really effective for loosening the hips. Men don't generally have loose hips, which has been clinically proven at wedding parties the world over. While still seated in *dandasana*, place your hands at your sides. Inhale, fill your lungs, then exhale and walk your hands out in front of you on the floor to wherever your tightness is. Your spine should be straight as a yardstick. Inhale into the tightness and exhale to soften. No need to go any further forward, just stay where that tightness is and breathe into it. Surprise! Now you're in *paschimottanasana* and you didn't even know it. Stay there for a few yoga breaths, then walk your hands back and sit up.

THE NOT-SO-BAD AND THE UGLY
Less forward bend. The not-so-bad?
Somewhere in between.

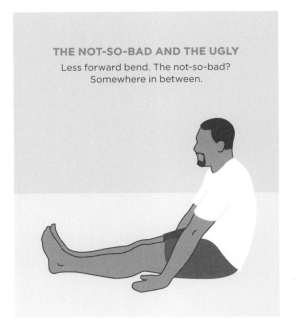

Cobbler's Pose (*Badda Konasana*) with Forward Bend

In most conventional yoga classes, you'd sit on the floor for the cobbler's pose. Jerry tells us to sit on a bolster or block. This is the third in a series of poses for loosening the hips. Men and that hip thing again. We're tight there. Also in the groin area. You know what I mean. This pose, in fact, is good for the midsection area in general.

Now that you're sitting on the bolster, position the soles of your feet together, hips splayed out to each side. There you go: really good splaying. Your knees should be higher than your hip crease (the joint between your upper thigh and hip). Position your thigh muscles so your pelvis is level. Think of your pelvis as a bowl of water you don't want to spill. As the crown of your head reaches toward the ceiling, drop your shoulders down.

Once more, grab a block, or try a telephone book. Actually, who has those anymore? That full box of Wheaties will suffice. With cereal box (or whatever) between both palms, hold your arms out straight in front of you. Then rotate them up to twelve-o'clock high, until your outstretched arms are back by your ears. Use your slow, calm breath.

Keeping this posture, bring your arms down and put the block/Wheaties box aside. Lastly, take your thumbs and index fingers and hook them around each big toe, right hand to right foot, left to left. Jerry at this point helpfully recommends rubbing your elbows into your thighs to maintain an outward rotation of the pelvis. Inhale, and on the exhale, lean forward with a flat spine until you reach your tight spot. Breathe into that tightness and on the exhale, see if it softens. Don't go any further forward. Stay there even if the tightness goes away. Breathe.

THE GOOD

If you can bend a bit, demote yourself to a blanket or the floor.

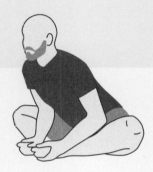

THE NOT-SO-BAD AND THE UGLY

On a bolster, minimal bend. Split the difference and you've got the not-so-bad.

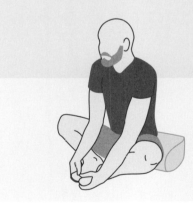

Wide Angle Pose (*Upavistha*) with Forward Bend

Here's the fourth and final pose in the symmetrical pose series. It's called wide angle because that's the way your legs go: wide. You're basically going to imitate a turkey wishbone on Thanksgiving. But you're the lucky one. Nobody's going to try to pull you apart.

If you ever ran track, you might have performed a similar sort of stretch for those hurdling muscles. Except there's no running involved with this *asana*. You're already practically in position. Sit on a bolster or block. But this time keep your legs straight and bring them wide.

Relax: Nobody's expecting you to do the splits. Forming a V with your legs is enough. Just like everything else in yoga, go only as far as you're comfortable. Don't be a hero. This isn't hero's pose—that's somewhere else in this book. It's *upavistha*. Don't strain. Engage your thigh muscles by pressing the back of your knees down to the floor. That's more important than how much you can spread your legs (I'm not even going to stoop to make a joke about that; Yoga Matt's totally PG).

Just like you've done three times already, grab a block and hold it in your palms with your arms in front of you. Next, rotate your shoulders until your hands are above your head. Breathe. That's such a good idea, do it again.

Bring your arms down and place the block aside. Inhale, and on the exhale, bend forward until you locate your stopping point. Don't try to bend further or round your back to get lower. Instead, try to loosen the tightness by breathing. Remain in the forward bend for a few measured yoga breaths. Now you should be completely symmetrical. Well, maybe except for your hair.

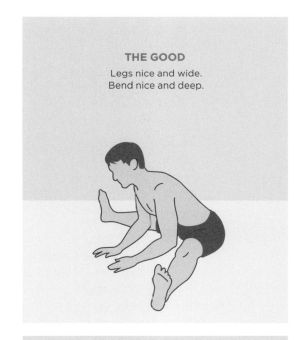

THE GOOD
Legs nice and wide.
Bend nice and deep.

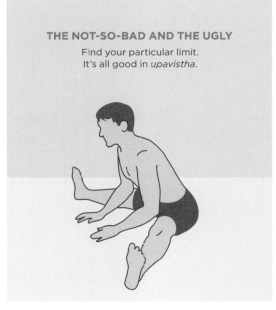

THE NOT-SO-BAD AND THE UGLY
Find your particular limit.
It's all good in *upavistha*.

Downward Dog (*Adho Mukha Svanasana*), Modified

Here's a new breed of downward dog. Instead of performing it on all fours like, well, a dog, we're including the extra equipment of a chair and wall. The reason? Men are often tight in their hamstrings. We're runners, cyclists, leg pressers of incredible sums of weight. The addition of a chair and wall make this a more comfortable and man-friendly pose. It's about time, isn't it, that somebody thought of us?

The chair also alleviates pressure on the wrists, a common obstacle for beginners, or pups in the case of downward dog. It's good for people with lower back pain, too. Begin by placing the back chair legs firmly against the wall so that the chair can support your weight. Stand in front of the chair and grab the corners of the chair seat, one hand at each corner, wedged in the meat of your palm. Then step your feet back until your body forms a hinge at the waist. Roughly, your body should resemble the gable of a house, a roof of straight legs and straight back, your heinie the crown of the roof.

The key for any version of downward dog is to maintain a long spine, like a dachshund. If you need to bend your legs a little or lift your heels off the floor, you're not

---

JERRY SAYS

"One of my teachers used to say about yoga, 'Try to take the inside out and outside in.' I'm pretty sure he wasn't talking about food."

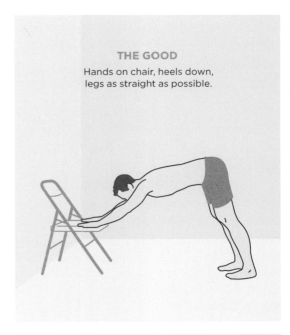

THE GOOD

Hands on chair, heels down,
legs as straight as possible.

a bad dog. It's perfectly okay. Good dog. Try pulling your kneecaps up toward your waist. Now relax your neck and let your head hang down. Hold for five long yoga breaths. Then walk your feet back to the chair and slowly roll up to standing.

Once you become a downward dog fancier, here are some tasty tips:

1. Make sure you use a sturdy chair.

2. If you're a guest, ask your host if it's okay to put the chair to that use.

3. Bark only in the privacy of your own home.

4. Resist the urge to lift your leg. It's not funny. This is *adho mukha svanasana*, after all.

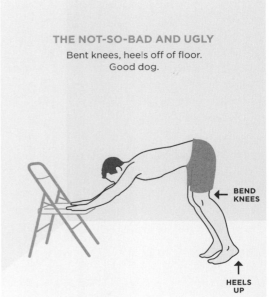

THE NOT-SO-BAD AND UGLY

Bent knees, heels off of floor.
Good dog.

← BEND KNEES

↑ HEELS UP

Mountain Pose (Tadasana) and Forward Fold (Uttanasana)

The sun salutation is a very traditional yoga practice. Many people perform it first thing in the day, to greet the rising sun. Kind of yoga's version of a gentle eye-opener.

Begin in mountain pose (*tadasana*). Stand up tall with toes touching or slightly apart, but with the outsides of your feet parallel, heels a little separated. Breathe with an open chest, hands at your side, palms facing forward. Inhale and look up with only your eyes (without tipping your head back or raising your shoulders). Exhale and return to looking straight ahead. Perform this three times. (Remember my handy-dandy mnemonic device for mountain pose: To the tune of "It's Impossible": It's *tadasana*, when you stand there with your arms at your sides, it's just *tadasana*.)

JERRY SAYS

"When breathing during these *asanas,* try to imagine a thin tube from your mouth extending down to your pubic bone. Fill the tube in both directions with an even flow. If you're panting, you're pushing the pose too far."

The third time Jerry incorporates a forward fold, like a mini nap right in the middle of the *asana.* Here's how it works: First, your blocks. They should be at your sides near your feet, positioned on end at their highest level. Exhale and bend at the waist, hands to the blocks. Simply bend forward and relax with your head near your knees and chill for a couple of breaths. Bend your knees a little if you like; it's called resting. Inhale and look up with a flat back. Exhale and fold back down. Inhale and roll up to *tadasana.*

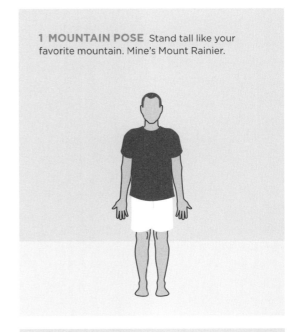

1 MOUNTAIN POSE Stand tall like your favorite mountain. Mine's Mount Rainier.

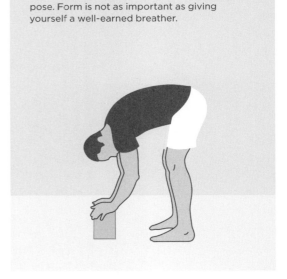

2 FORWARD FOLD Considered a resting pose. Form is not as important as giving yourself a well-earned breather.

Chair Pose (Utkatanasana) with a Twist (Parivrtta Utkatanasana)

32

We're still technically in Jerry's flow-ing sun salutation. He throws just about everything in there except for the kitchen sink. This is where Jerry adds the chair pose to the mix. Don't get your hopes up. It doesn't involve a real chair.

Begin in upright mountain pose, stand-ing up straight with your hands at your sides, palms open and facing forward, arm and leg muscles engaged. Big toes are together, the outside edges of the feet parallel while keeping a little space between your heels. Inhale. On your exhale, pretend like you're sitting, bending your knees with arms stretched out and up alongside your ears—that old yogi ver-sion of *touchdown!* Make sure your weight is balanced over your heels. This isn't squat pose. It's chair pose. Try to look like a chair you might want to sit in: balanced with a nice, straight back.

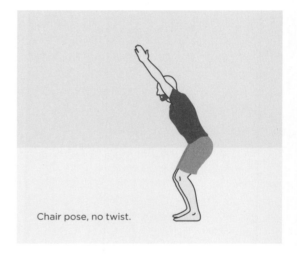

Chair pose, no twist.

Remain in chair pose for a few calm breaths. Then exhale and, using your core muscles, rise back up into mountain pose. Repeat the entire movement two more times.

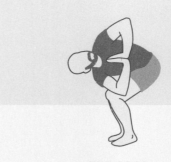

THE GOOD

Big bend in the knees. The twistiest
of twists with the top shoulder pointing up
to the ceiling. Eyes gazing up, too.

Before we're done, Jerry likes to add a twist. Assume chair pose once more—outsides of the feet parallel, knees bent, arms stretched up alongside the ears. Next, place your right elbow outside your left knee and gaze toward the left side of the room. Breathe in place. Your other side of the body then gets to twist, with your left elbow outside your right knee while you peer at that spot on the wall on the right side of the room. Breathe in, breathe out. Untwist and then roll back up into mountain pose. If elbows outside the knee is too much, your hand is enough.

Terrific job. But the sun hasn't quite set. The next pose is still part of Jerry's summer solstice longest-day-of-the-year sun salutation.

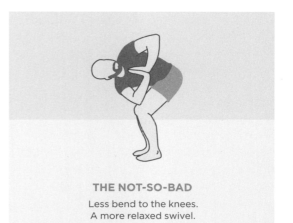

THE NOT-SO-BAD

Less bend to the knees.
A more relaxed swivel.

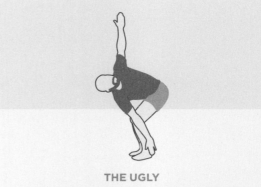

THE UGLY

Minimal knee bend. Less twist, use a steadying
arm. Kind of the stool version of chair pose.

Lunge to Pyramid Pose (Parsvottanasana)

Have two blocks handy, one on either side of you. We're going to build a pyramid. Intense side stretch is another description of this pose.

Begin in mountain pose. Widen your stance to hip-width. As a guide, place two fists side by side down between your feet. Step back with your right leg. With your hands on the blocks, bend your front leg to a 90-degree angle and do a lunge. Your front knee should be directly over your ankle, not past it. Your back foot is on its toes, and your toes are pointing forward. Do a little back bend, looking up. If you can manage it, raise your arms up toward the ceiling. Repeat on the other side.

Next, do the lunge with your right leg back again, hands on the blocks, and this time, from the lunge, straighten your front leg so that your two legs form an upside-down V. Drop your back heel to the floor and turn the toes of your back foot out at roughly 45 degrees. Keep your hips squared forward. Rather than heel-arch

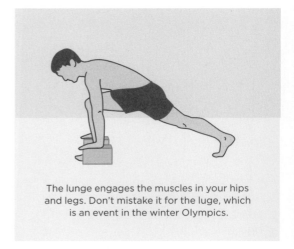

The lunge engages the muscles in your hips and legs. Don't mistake it for the luge, which is an event in the winter Olympics.

alignment, assume a wider stance, with your back foot more to the edge of your mat.

Try to keep both legs straight. Square your hips so your torso is facing forward, poised over your legs. Inhale and bend forward on the exhale, placing your hands on the blocks on either side of you. The most important thing is to keep your front leg straight. How much you can bend forward is secondary. As you inhale, imagine you're calmly filling a thin pipe that extends all the way down to your pelvis. Exhale slowly, and refill again. The stretch extends from your hamstrings all the way up to your shoulders. This *asana* is also aces for balance.

Jerry always says, "When you get really good at this, you can place your hands on the floor instead of the blocks and even bend your elbows." (Then he tells us about some beachfront real estate he'd like to sell in Florida.)

To come out of this pose, use your core muscles to pull yourself back up to a standing position. You can remember to do that by reaching up as if you're grabbing air and use your abs to climb into mountain pose.

Before you dismantle that pyramid, the other side gets the same stretch. Left leg goes back to form the upside-down V. Drop the back heel to the floor and turn your back foot out at a 45-degree angle. Hands go to the blocks. Keeping a straight front leg is job number one. Bending forward so your body describes a pyramid is secondary to that. Don't overdo it. Find what Jerry calls "your edge," that final point of stretching before it begins to hurt.

Last, pull yourself back up to mountain pose by relying on your core. Both of your sides should feel equally cooked.

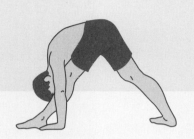

THE GOOD

Legs wide apart. Hands on floor. Both legs straight. You've solved the mystery of the pyramid.

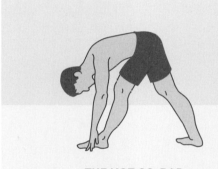

THE NOT-SO-BAD

Legs not so wide, maybe bent a little. Only the fingertips touching the floor.

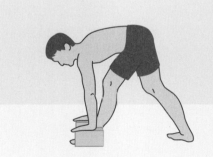

THE UGLY

Hands on blocks. A mild forward bend. Legs closer together. Knees a little bent. Remember to breathe. This will all be over soon.

Warrior 1 (Virabhadrasana 1)

Can you believe we're still in Jerry's extended sunrise salutation? Warrior 1 is the next pose that we segue into from mountain pose (*tadasana*). Now that you're properly oriented, step back with your left leg, about three or four feet. Bend your front knee so that shin and thigh form a 90-degree angle. You want your knee over your ankle. Drop your back heel and rotate your toes outward 45 degrees. Just as before, your rear foot will be in a wider stance.

For the more balance-challenged, such as *moi*, move your left foot out to the left a bit to achieve more stability and a more solid base. Whichever you choose, keep your hips straight and facing forward. It's a big point in warrior 1.

Once your hips are square and aimed toward the front of the room, raise your arms up by your ears. Maintain that long, measured breath just like a warrior would.

Then bring your arms down and step forward into mountain pose. Or take several steps back into mountain, which is less of a strain.

JERRY SAYS

"Your balance changes daily. Sometimes I can do this all day long. Others, it's like, whoa, too much wine or something."

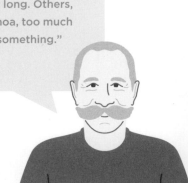

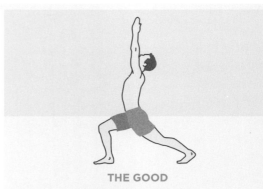

THE GOOD
Arms straight up by ears.
Eyes are studying the ceiling overhead.
Your back has a slight arch.

Before we move on, you have your right side to do. So step back with your right foot and bend the left knee. Angle your right toes out for some more stability. Move your foot wider if you need a more solid base. Last, reach those arms up.

To finish warrior 1, step forward with your trailing right leg back into mountain pose. Breathe.

Just because I give a capsule review of the *asana* in the second half isn't an invitation to rush things. Both sides get equal treatment. If you need to, before you get fluent in these poses, just gaze up a few paragraphs to glean the finer points. I'm merely trying not to repeat myself unnecessarily, which Yoga Matt's wife, Beth Matt, says he does all the time.

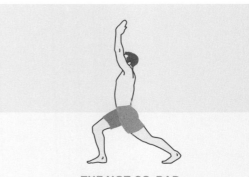

THE NOT-SO-BAD
Arms not as straight up.
Looking forward. No arch in back.

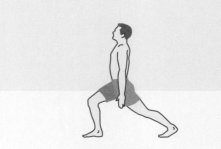

THE UGLY
Arms at sides. Make sure those hips are squared. Fiercely hold your ground. This is warrior 1, *not* worrier 1.

Warrior 2 (Virabhadrasana 2)

Finally, the end of Jerry's jack-of-all-trades sun salutation. From the last *asana*, warrior 1, we flow into warrior 2. The big differentiating factor between these fierce stances is the hips. Unlike warrior 1, in warrior 2 your hips will face toward the side of the room because, as anyone in the army can tell you, danger comes from all directions.

Besides fending off potential enemies, warrior 2 is an effective stretch for keeping your ankles, knees, groin, and hips in fine fighting form. It's good for stamina, too, especially when you hold the pose for multiple breaths.

This last leg of Jerry's sunny journey begins in mountain pose, which at this point can be summed up as standing tall with your arms at your sides. Step back with your left leg. Bend your front (right) knee so that your upper and lower leg form a 90-degree angle. Your knee

should be directly over your ankle, not behind or in front of it—especially not in front of it, which is murder on the knees. Drop your back heel as in the previous *asana* and turn your toes out 45 degrees. If you can, aim for a heel-arch alignment

JERRY SAYS

"There are three different warrior poses, each good for balance. Especially warrior 2, which Yoga Matt insists on calling the surfer 2. I used to surf. He might have a point."

between your front and back feet. For a more solid base, position your back foot a bit more to the left.

In warrior 2, keep your hips and torso facing the left side of the room. Bring your arms up so they're parallel to the floor, right arm forward, left arm back, with palms down. Gaze forward, out over the fingers of your right hand. Hold this pose for a few breaths. In Hawaii, they call this surfer 2 (just kidding). Then step back into mountain pose.

Your other side gets the same basic training. From mountain pose, step back with your right leg. Bend your front, left leg at 90 degrees, knee over ankle. In any version of warrior, your knee should *never* go beyond that 90-degree point so it's out in front of your foot.

Next, drop the back heel, toes out 45 degrees, relying on a wider stance if needed. Are your hips and torso aimed toward the right side of the room? Good. Now bring your arms up parallel to the floor, palms down. Gaze over your left hand.

Enjoy a few yoga breaths in the pose, then step back into mountain pose. Congratulations, Jerry's sun salutation has officially set.

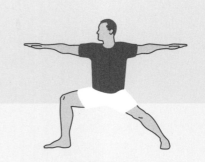

THE GOOD
Heel-arch alignment is in place.
A deep bend in the front leg. Distance front to back between feet on mat is wide.

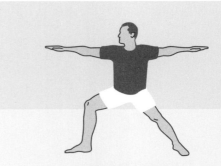

THE NOT-SO-BAD
Back foot is out to the side.
A gentler bend to the front leg, shorter distance between your feet.

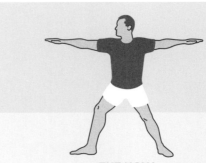

THE UGLY
Less distance between feet front to back.
The angle of front knee doesn't have to be 90 degrees. For a little more troop backup, perform warrior 2 against the wall.

Wrap-Up

Here's the big circle of Jerry's sun salutation, a foundational sequence in yoga where you flow from pose to pose. The center is you in *tadasana*, the spokes of the wheel attached to each pose. You start in mountain pose and return to it after each successive *asana*. Study this closely. It will definitely be on the test.

1 MOUNTAIN POSE Uses every muscle in the body and helps reduce back pain.

2 FORWARD FOLD Calming and rejuvenating.

3 CHAIR POSE Strengthens the thighs and ankles.

4 LUNGE Opens hips and chest; stretches the groin and legs.

5 PYRAMID POSE Stretches the hamstrings.

6 WARRIOR 1 Strengthens and stretches the legs and opens the chest. Develops concentration and balance. Energizing.

7 WARRIOR 2 Strengthens legs, opens hips and chest. Improves circulation and energizes the body.

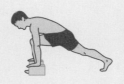

4 LUNGE

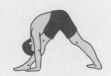

5 PYRAMID POSE

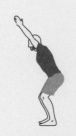

3 CHAIR POSE

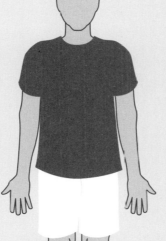

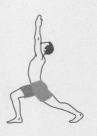

6 WARRIOR 1

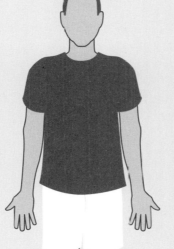

2 FORWARD FOLD

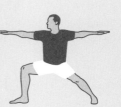

7 WARRIOR 2

1 MOUNTAIN POSE

Balancing and Tree Pose (*Vrksasana*)

Men and good balance don't always go together. We have higher centers of gravity than women. Face it, we're tippy. This series of poses is useful for enhancing balance and stretching the inner thigh and groin. Anything that safely stretches the groin—you know it has to be good for you.

Start in mountain pose (*tadasana*): Feet together, outsides of feet parallel with a little space between your heels, weight evenly distributed over both feet.

Lift your kneecaps and engage your thigh muscles. Your arms should be at your sides with open palms facing out in front of you. Reach the crown of your head toward the ceiling while allowing your shoulders to drop. Keep a calm and steady breath.

Now shift your weight to your right foot and place your left foot in front of your right, heel to toe. Find your balance and close your eyes. Breathe. With eyes

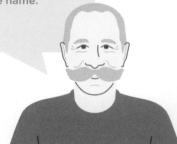

JERRY SAYS

"Sometimes during a pose it helps to focus on a fixed point, which is called a *drishti*. I think I once dated a girl back in the '70s with the same name."

closed, you might waver in place a bit like a perp in a drunken driving field test. That's okay. Nobody's going to arrest you. Just remember to breathe.

Repeat this movement on the other side, with the weight on your left foot, right foot in front. Find your balance and close your eyes. People (that includes men) frequently have better balance on one side or the other, which is as natural as righties and lefties.

Here comes the tree part. You can do this with one hand on a wall, if needed, to maintain balance. With your weight on your right foot, raise your left foot up so your knee is pointing out to the side like a triangle. Rest your foot on your right ankle, calf, or thigh, *but never at the knee* (your knee's a joint; don't put sideways pressure on the hinge). You can also use your left foot as a prop, with your toes on the floor and the sole of your left foot against your right ankle. Lift your arms toward the ceiling but keep your shoulders down. If raised arms cause you to wobble, bring your palms together in front of your chest.

Repeat with the other foot. Here, too, your sense of balance might vary. All perfectly normal, so long as you remember to breathe.

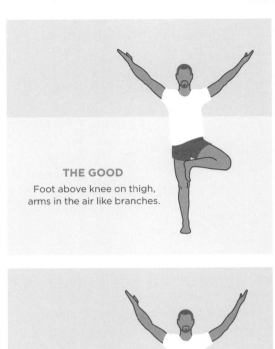

THE GOOD
Foot above knee on thigh,
arms in the air like branches.

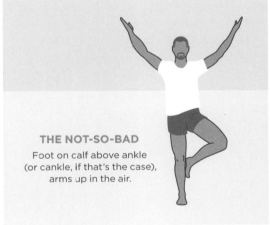

THE NOT-SO-BAD
Foot on calf above ankle
(or cankle, if that's the case),
arms up in the air.

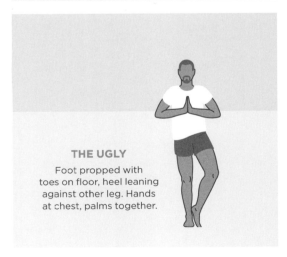

THE UGLY
Foot propped with
toes on floor, heel leaning
against other leg. Hands
at chest, palms together.

Pelvic Tilts

Hey, Elvis, this involves your pelvis. All you have to do is lie on your back on your mat with legs out straight. Have a block handy to insert in the small of your back to alleviate strain at any time. So far this doesn't seem much like exercise, does it? Keeping your legs out straight, tip your pelvis forward, bringing the small of your back up off the floor. (In other words, stick your butt out.) Do this a couple more times. Basically, make like a fish on the sand in slow motion, except unlike a fish, remember to breathe.

Next, bend your knees and place your feet flat on the mat. Tilt forward and then back, lifting your pelvis off the mat, then landing your butt softly back on the matt. Repeat, tilting forward, then back, pelvis lifting off the mat. If you need the block, use it.

JERRY SAYS

"Using a block is a back saver. The yoga block is your stepping-stone to more advanced poses."

We're not done with that pelvis. Do all of the above except tilt up to the middle of your back. Return to earth slowly, then tilt forward and back, reaching the middle of your back once more, then down. Position the block under you to relieve strain, if necessary.

Last, tilt all the way up to your shoulder blades. Roll back down and tilt your pelvis forward, lifting the small of your back a skosh off the mat. Then do it back and forth again. If you prefer, you can do this last part with your feet closer on the mat to your butt. One more thing. Breathe.

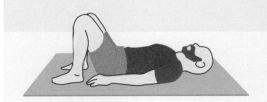

1 First things first, tilt your pelvis forward.

Then tilt your pelvis back. Make like your pelvis is a glass of water and you're pouring it forward and pouring it back.

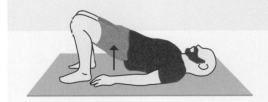

2 Next, tilt your pelvis to the middle of your back.

And last, if you can, tilt back all the way to your shoulder blades.

Leg Stretch

Stay on your back from the previous pose. In this stretch, you're essentially going to raise both legs up to twelve o'clock, then slowly lower them back down to the floor at nine o'clock. In Jerry's class, you're allowed to use a block under the sacrum—the triangular bone at the base of your spine between your hip bones and pelvis—to make this stretch less of a stretch for a guy. (We have tight hammies and calf muscles.)

"If at any time during the pose your back gets too tight," Jerry advises, **"bend your knees."** You already have a block deployed under your sacrum—you're in position. Jerry, what a genius. That's why they pay him the medium bucks for teaching this class.

Lift your right leg as though you're standing on the ceiling, ankle flexed, leg straight—or some reasonable facsimile of straight. Breathe in and out, then see if you can take your right heel back down to the mat with your leg straight. Repeat the same with your left leg. Again, try to bring your heel down gently to the mat. If need be, bend your knees to lower your legs.

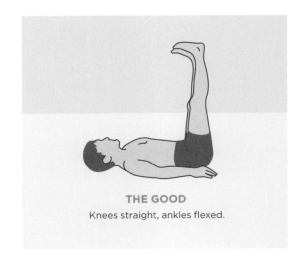

THE GOOD
Knees straight, ankles flexed.

Finally, "stand on the ceiling" with both legs up. (If there's any straining in your back, bend the knees.) Pause for a breath. Lower both heels down to the mat in tandem. Once you do, bend your knees with your feet on the floor. Lift the pelvis and pull the block out from underneath you. Now lower yourself down vertebra by vertebra. You can also do this raised up on your toes as you bring your back down to the mat in slow motion. Once you've returned to earth, place your feet wide and bring your bent knees together for some good old constructive rest. You earned it.

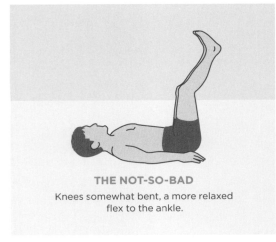

THE NOT-SO-BAD
Knees somewhat bent, a more relaxed flex to the ankle.

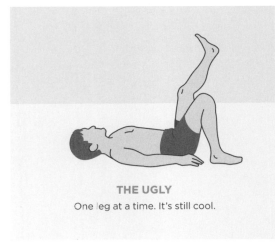

THE UGLY
One leg at a time. It's still cool.

Vishnu's Couch (*Anantasana*)

When I heard the name of this pose, I thought it was right up my alley. Sorry, no couch. I wonder what this Vishnu guy calls a table.

Instead of a couch, have a strap handy and lie on your right side with your back against the wall. Make like a wall yourself: the entire length of your body should be in contact with the vertical surface. Bend your right elbow so your hand can bear the weight of your head to eliminate neck strain. Using the wall to maintain alignment, bend your left leg, and with your left hand, put the strap under your foot. Now straighten your left leg up toward the ceiling while continuing to hold the ends of the strap in your left hand. See if you can straighten your left arm, too. You'll have to adjust where you grip the strap to do this.

"Eventually," Jerry always promises us, "you won't need to use the strap or the wall." Yeah, right. Jerry also claims that in lieu of the strap, with a straight arm, you'll hook your left index finger around your left big toe. Until that magical day, using the strap is just fine. Just make sure in this pose that your outstretched leg is making full contact with the wall.

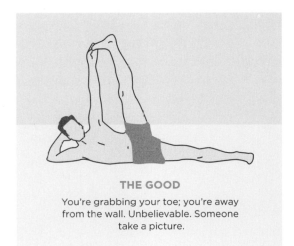

THE GOOD

You're grabbing your toe; you're away from the wall. Unbelievable. Someone take a picture.

To come out of this pose, bend your knee and slide the strap off your foot. Then repeat the process on your other side. Once you do that, lie on your back for some well-earned constructive rest.

Jerry suggests watching TV this way because Vishnu's couch is a great *asana* for your oblique muscles and your hamstrings, not to mention your groin. I don't think I'm ever going over to his house to catch a football game.

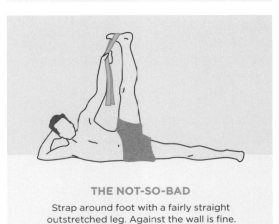

THE NOT-SO-BAD

Strap around foot with a fairly straight outstretched leg. Against the wall is fine.

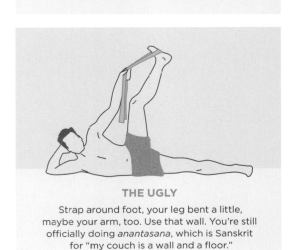

THE UGLY

Strap around foot, your leg bent a little, maybe your arm, too. Use that wall. You're still officially doing *anantasana*, which is Sanskrit for "my couch is a wall and a floor."

Windshield Wipers

And now, a brief respite after Vishnu's couch. Here are some words you're going to like hearing: lie on your back on your mat with your knees bent.

Gently bring your tented legs all the way down to the right side of the mat, orienting your left knee over your right ankle. Reach your left arm up over your head. Stretch and breathe before your arm returns to your side. Next, slowly bring your knees back up and gently lower them to the left side of the mat and reach up over your head with your right arm. Then do your other side again, nice and slow.

JERRY SAYS

"Remember: Your windows aren't done until you do a diagonal stretch on both sides."

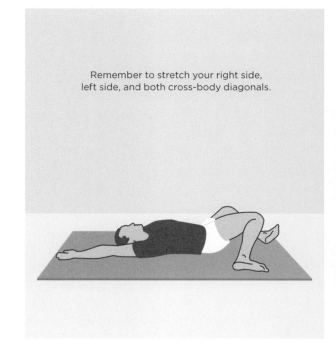

Remember to stretch your right side, left side, and both cross-body diagonals.

Go back and forth, right leg, left leg, opposite arm extending on the floor above your head. To a fly on the ceiling you should kind of look like windshield wipers, with your arms sweeping up toward your ears.

Then, before you're done, do a couple of reps with your right arm, right leg to the mat and left arm, left leg to the mat, rather than opposing limbs. Okay, your windows should be clean.

Resting Pose (*Savasana*) and Breathing in Thirds

Savasana is the first yoga pose for which yours truly, your faithful guide, Yoga Matt, bothered to learn the traditional Sanskrit name. You'll know you're pronouncing it correctly if it includes the sound *aaaah*.

This is the reward after an hour of contorting your body on a sticky mat. Consider this a necessary interval to relax after an exercise session, rather than rushing off to the next thing in your day. Men are particularly prone to this syndrome. Antsy, constantly looking ahead, impatient.

Well, slow down, cowboy. There are many roads that lead to *savasana*. You can do an inversion, such as legs up the wall (page 80). Or lie on your back, with a folded blanket under your head, a bolster under your knees, feet wide. Charlie Chaplin feet are okay.

According to Jerry, *savasana* is the second most important part of the yoga practice—the need after exertion to make an equal and opposite noneffort. Gee, it sounds tough. If you say so, Jerry.

In order to stay in the here and now, we perform a breathing cadence called third breaths. Start by inhaling all the way down to the pelvis, the first third, and pause. Don't exhale yet. Then continue to inhale into the second third, the next shelf up,

JERRY SAYS

"Some people call racing thoughts *monkey mind*. I call it the whirligig. The thing you need to take a step back from every once in a while. Use *savasana* as often as needed."

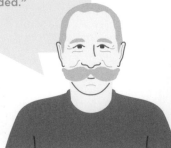

in the diaphragm area, and pause once more. For the *third* third, breathe in all the way up to the chest and throat like you're filling a glass of water. To exhale, open the mouth and let all three thirds out. Then do the whole series of breathing three more times.

After your final round of third breaths, continue to lie on your mat, inhaling more gently through your nose, letting the exhale float out of your mouth without any noise. If your mind wanders or you find yourself distracted, return to this unhurried, measured breathing cadence.

To reemerge from *savasana*, take a fuller, deeper breath. Move the small muscles in your body, your fingers and toes. Reinhabit your body from the bottom up—feet, legs, pelvis, back, stomach, chest, shoulders, arms and hands, neck and head. Keep your eyes closed as long as you can. Stay in your yoga state of mind.

To get up, bring your knees toward your chest, roll to your right, and stay down there for a few breaths to allow your blood pressure to level off. Then turn and face the floor. Perform a modified push-up and sit cross-legged on the floor. Now put your palms together, fingers separated, thumbs to chest. See if you can bring your chin to your chest without collapsing your chest down. Good. Next comes the part where you say *namaste*.

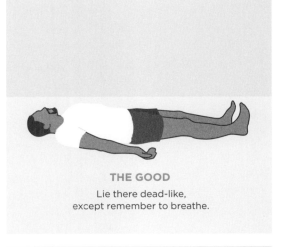

THE GOOD
Lie there dead-like,
except remember to breathe.

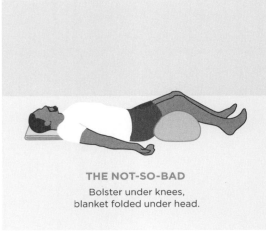

THE NOT-SO-BAD
Bolster under knees,
blanket folded under head.

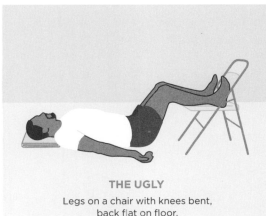

THE UGLY
Legs on a chair with knees bent,
back flat on floor.

MANLY YOGA PRACTICE NO. 2

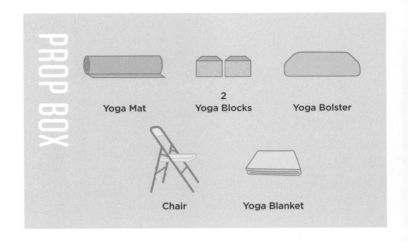

Yoga Mat

2 Yoga Blocks

Yoga Bolster

Chair

Yoga Blanket

Now that you've survived Manly Yoga Practice No. 1, we have a completely new bunch of poses to unkink the knots. Always allow for a three-day rest between yoga sessions. It's not twice-a-day summer practices on the high school football team. Your muscles need time to recover. Like all of Jerry's classes, this practice starts and ends with the breath. You're going to be doing legs up the wall and cat-cow, triangle, and half-moon poses. A veritable greatest hits of yoga.

There's still more. This second breed of downward dog introduced here? It helps promote increased focus and relieve insomnia. How about that seated forward bend? It might just make you smarter and help you better digest that pepperoni pizza you ate last night. And don't forget triangle pose, which is good for pains in the back of both metaphoric and physical origin.

For a few of the seated poses here, you might want to use a yoga block. With most seated poses, the correct posture is having the pelvic area above the knees. For those with tight hamstrings—most of us—that can be a strain, literally. The purpose of the block, therefore, is to raise the floor for your butt, which positions you in the proper vertical alignment.

This Manly Practice should take about an hour, just like the first. Remember, there's no such thing as speed yoga. A good rule of thumb is to ease into your point of resistance in each *asana*. Don't try to push through your limit. Rather, relax into it. Breathing helps. No gulping for air. Hold the pose for three to five rounds of measured yoga breaths. A few more cleansing breaths will prepare you for the next *asana*, then turn the page.

One last thing. Don't cheap out on *savasana*. Everything else can wait. This is where Jerry always says, "You worked hard in class today. Remember, this is your chance to make an equal and opposite noneffort." *Mmm*. Noneffort. Who doesn't like the sound of that?

Back Stretch with Bolster, Alternate Nostril Breathing

Jerry likes to start out with the breath as a focus because too often we, as humans, only breathe from our chest. Deeper, however, is more restorative and calming. A deep breath extends all the way down to your diaphragm.

I personally call this opening pose "couch potato on the floor." First, place a bolster lengthwise, propping a block under one end of the bolster so that the bolster's at an angle. You can place the block at whatever angle of repose you prefer. Now just lie back on the bolster, arms a little away from your sides—not too close or too far—palms facing toward the ceiling.

Pretty nice, this breathing stuff, huh? According to Jerry, breathing and yoga forever go together, like ham and mustard. As you're lying there, place your thumb on one nostril, and your ring finger on the other. Block one nostril with your thumb and inhale through the other nostril. Then block that nostril with your ring finger and unblock the other nostril and breathe out

JERRY SAYS

"They say it's not yoga unless you have your breath and it's not breath unless you have your yoga. I've been doing yoga for over twenty years and I'm not quite sure what the second half of that means."

and then in. Switch nostrils with your hand again. You'll get the hang of it. Basically, you're breathing out and in on one nostril, then out and in on the other. Do four cycles of this, nice and slow.

After the fourth round of alternate nostril breathing, put your arms back down at your sides. Inhale through your nose and let your exhale flow smoothly out through your mouth, Jerry's "slow, steady breath." He also says to imagine a long tube extending from your mouth to your pubic bone. Really, it's just a reminder to inhale calmly all the way down to your center. This is the breath to use during each *asana*. If you're straining or tensing up, ease back a bit. Calm and pleasurable rather than huffing and puffing. In fact, huffing and puffing is a sign of straining. Yoga's not "no pain, no gain." It's simply no pain, no pain. (I know—said before. I couldn't come up with a better rhyme. The only other option I have is "no injury, no perjury.")

Now that you've got your yoga breath going, move the props to the side and lie back down on the mat, gazing up at the ceiling. We usually spend the rest of the hour this way. Just kidding! Jerry's got a whole bunch of ways to make you more limber and wiser in Manly Yoga Practice No. 2.

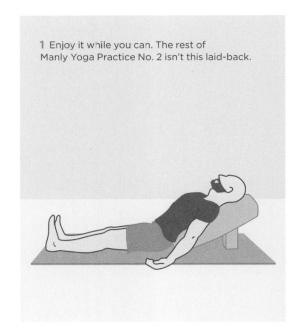

1 Enjoy it while you can. The rest of Manly Yoga Practice No. 2 isn't this laid-back.

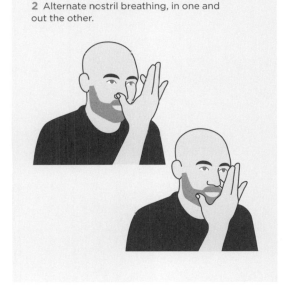

2 Alternate nostril breathing, in one and out the other.

Sphinx (*Salamba Bhujangasana*)

This pose is called *salamba bhujangasana*, a name as inscrutable as the mythological sphinx, but lucky for you, Jerry takes all the mystery out of the *asana*.

Lie down on your belly. Before you get all sphinxlike, we're going to stretch each side. Reach your arms out in front of you as if you're flying like Superman, and stretch. Get that nice long stretch going, with a little more focus on the left side extending all the way down your leg. Do the same with the right side of your body. Then stretch equally on both sides of the body, arms reaching forward, both legs reaching back, keeping the tops of your feet on the floor.

Here comes the sphinx part. Drag your hands back toward your body on the mat until your elbows are directly beneath your shoulders. Palms are on the floor. Lift your torso and head up while keeping your elbows on the mat. Lean into the left hand, then the right, and stretch your legs all the way straight back. The tops of your feet should be flush against the floor, and don't curl your toes.

Besides *salamba bhujangasana* and sphinx, this pose is also known as a baby backbend because it doesn't require any extreme torquing of the body. You're totally supported by the floor, baby! So it relieves stress without stressing the body.

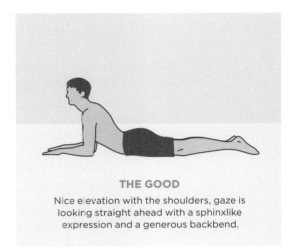

THE GOOD

Nice elevation with the shoulders, gaze is looking straight ahead with a sphinxlike expression and a generous backbend.

Hold the sphinx pose for five of Jerry's "long, steady breaths," then lower your chest back down to the mat. Do the sphinx pose again, rising up with your elbows under your shoulders, make like a statue for a few seconds, and then bring your chest back down.

A common error when performing *salamba bhujangasana* is a natural tendency to clench your butt muscles, which stresses the lower back—not the purpose of this pose. Don't clench the butt. It's probably good advice in general.

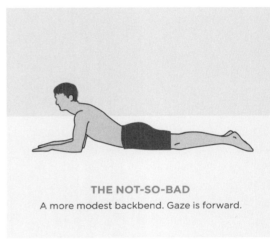

THE NOT-SO-BAD

A more modest backbend. Gaze is forward.

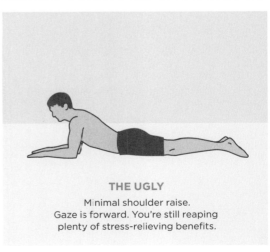

THE UGLY

Minimal shoulder raise.
Gaze is forward. You're still reaping plenty of stress-relieving benefits.

Locust (Salabhasana)

The locust pose is a nice back-to-back segue after the sphinx because it further loosens up the spine and opens up the chest. Thankfully, Jerry doesn't go full locust on you. This is a gentle version of *salabhasana*.

Assume the same belly-to-floor position as the sphinx. Bring your arms back toward your feet and clasp your hands behind your back. They should be hovering, roughly speaking, above your butt. Jerry likes to point his index fingers, but that's not compulsory. With arms stretching back, see if you can raise them a little higher over your back while lifting your chest off the mat. Hold for a few yoga breaths and then lower yourself back down to the mat. Rest with one cheek on the mat.

Next, your arms go back again as before, but this time switch out the orientation, with your opposite little finger on the bottom of your clasped hands. It should feel a little different because we tend to have a dominant side (except for yours truly, Yoga Matt, who's ambidextrous and can't tell his right from his left without remembering which hand he uses to salute the flag).

Lift your arms in this position as before and bring your chest up. While you're elevated, lift your right shoulder and look at the ceiling, but leave your pelvis on the ground. You should be leaning somewhat to the left. Breathe a few yoga breaths and return to neutral. Your left shoulder is next. Lift it and look up at the ceiling as before, leaning to the right with your pelvis on the mat, hold the pose for a few seconds, and then return to neutral. Bring your arms to your sides, and one cheek (your choice) to the mat. Take a few moments to rest.

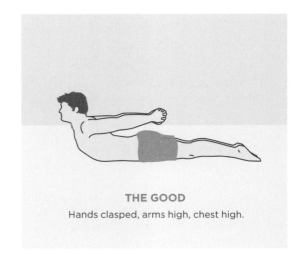

THE GOOD
Hands clasped, arms high, chest high.

Sometimes when we do this *asana*, Jerry instructs us to lift the "eyes" of our shoulders toward the ceiling. I don't know about Jerry's anatomy, but I don't have any eyes in my shoulders. It's really what writers who graduate from fancy MFA programs (not me) call a metaphor. Jerry's talking about that ho low nestled between your shoulder blade and the rotator cuff. Imagine there's an eye there and you're directing its focus to the ceiling. This helps you open up your chest muscles down through your rib cage. Good for breathing and showing off that manly chest.

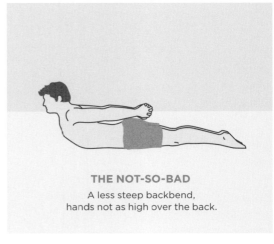

THE NOT-SO-BAD
A less steep backbend,
hands not as high over the back.

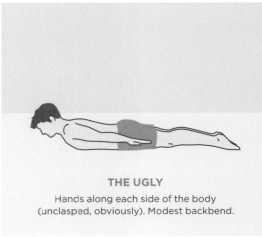

THE UGLY
Hands along each side of the body
(unclasped, obviously). Modest backbend.

Cat-Cow (Marjaryasana-Bitilasana)

This combination of poses is like a science fiction movie because a cat turns into a cow and back again, over and over. The method behind Jerry's madness is to do a bit more stretching before we dive into the more vigorous portion of the practice that follows.

Get on all fours, resting on your hands and knees. Here's the important part: let your tailbone do the leading. I know, I know. It's like one of the few times in life it's okay to lead with your butt. Make sure first, though, that your hands are under your shoulders, knees about hip-width apart. Tuck your tailbone, round your back, and then drop your head. In case you couldn't tell, that's a drop-dead imitation of a cat.

From here you're going to gradually evolve into a cow. Lift the tailbone and sag down into the cow pose by dropping your belly and having your head follow by looking up (it's sort of an *inward* arch). Moo: you're a cow.

The transition back and forth between the two poses should be smooth and slow. Jerry always stretches out the "baaaaack and forth," like he's talking to a child or someone from a foreign country. Then Jerry likes to dress up the cat and cow a bit. If it's too much for you—or too confusing—stick with the classic movement described above.

JERRY SAYS

"Use your hindquarters to lead in cat–cow. The rest of your body follows like a rope."

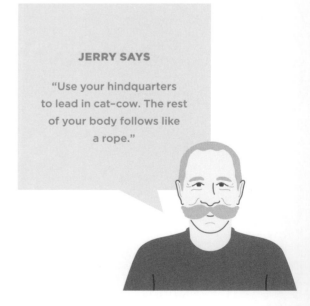

Begin the cat pose, dropping the tailbone, arching the back, head descending last. Except as you drop the tailbone, push your hips back at the same time, so you are sitting on your haunches. Now you turn into a cow. You're going to push your hips forward at the same time as you lift your tailbone and sag your gut. You're still moving forward as fluidly as a runny nose, continuing to drop your tailbone until your pelvis is on the floor. Then look up like a cow in a field before you begin to flow back into cat by lifting your pelvis back up and bringing your hips rearward as you drop your tailbone. Arch your back and you're once again a cat on its haunches. Check out the diagram (bottom) to catch the whole movement.

It's kind of a dance step, like the funky chicken, except it's the funkfied cat-cow. Practice a little to find your rhythm. Once you do, repeat a few times, like you can't decide whether you're a cat or a cow. Remember, if this more complicated version is too taxing or as confusing as the dance chart to the mamba, do the basic cat and cow. The variation is a nod to Vinyasa yoga, which uses flowing sequences between poses accompanied by regulated breathing. Whichever flavor you choose, come back to neutral on all fours at the end.

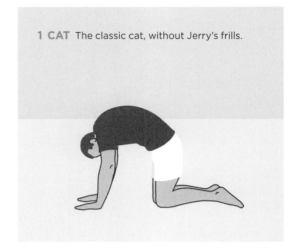

1 CAT The classic cat, without Jerry's frills.

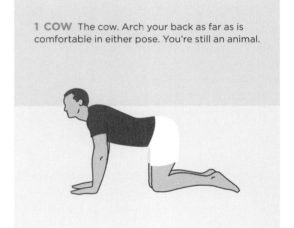

1 COW The cow. Arch your back as far as is comfortable in either pose. You're still an animal.

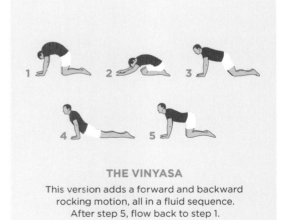

THE VINYASA
This version adds a forward and backward rocking motion, all in a fluid sequence. After step 5, flow back to step 1.

Shoulder Stretch (*Parsva Balasana*)

This is for all the guys out there who lift things, play sports, and have tight upper bodies in general. Pretty much all of us. We men are reachers and hefters. This *asana* should help with this particular difficulty of being a man.

Begin on all fours, knees and hands supporting you. Remember to breathe like a normal human being. Inhale and reach your left hand up to the ceiling, then look up at your left hand. As you exhale, sweep the arm down in front of your body and between your right arm and knee. Extend your left arm, as if forming half of a cross, bringing your left shoulder and cheek to the floor. As an option, use a blanket or bolster to prop your head up. Your left arm should be stretching outward from the trunk of your body in a perpendicular-ish fashion, palm up. To take the stretch a little further, reach your right leg back behind you.

It's okay to stop right there. But if you're feeling good, put your right arm behind you as if you're a speed skater or servant on *Downton Abbey*. Aim your right shoulder at the ceiling. Maintain your balance. More? No problem. Providing you have the balance, extend your right arm toward the ceiling. (Please note diagram. The previous description might suggest an act that's illegal in several states, including Mississippi.) Extend the stretch all the way to your fingertips. Breathe, then bring your right hand back to the mat and move your left arm so you come back to neutral on all fours.

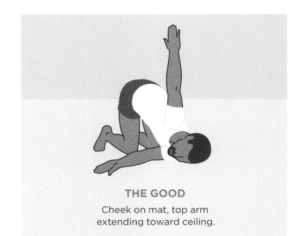

THE GOOD
Cheek on mat, top arm
extending toward ceiling.

Repeat with the right arm and remember to breathe. Perform two or three repetitions, alternating arms Hold the final stretch for five relaxed yoga breaths. Once you master the shoulder stretch, here are a few handy tips:

1. Make sure the mat is clean before you apply your face to it.

2. Probably more of an at-home than public type of pose.

3. But if you do choose to perform the pose in public and someone asks you what the heck you're doing, tell them *parsva balasana*.

4. As with all of these exercises, it's good to come into the practice with a basic understanding of right and left.

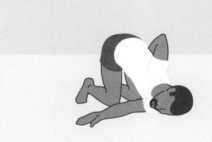

THE NOT-SO-BAD
Cheek on mat, top arm behind back.

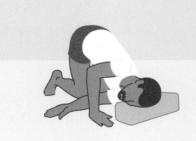

THE UGLY
Cheek on bolster, left arm on floor through the opening between your right arm and knee.

Triangle Pose (*Trikonasana*) with Chair and Bolster

You need a chair for this pose. A simple folding one works best, but anything will do. Place the chair at the end of your mat so it doesn't slip; it should be positioned to your left, with the front feet at the edge, the back facing you. Don't get your hopes up. This *asana* doesn't involve sitting.

Place a yoga bolster upright on the back side of the chair seat. Take a quick glance at the illustrations for this pose. What's the deal with the chair and bolster? Trust me, your neck will thank you. The bolster on the chair provides excellent support for that big ol' tater on your shoulders.

Start with your left foot at the base of the chair, toes pointing forward. Step wide with your right foot and align your right arch with your left heel. Maintain this nice heel-arch alignment, and imagine there's a wall behind you, keeping you plumb. With your straight back against the "wall," lower your left shoulder downward as if there's a hinge at your waist. The rest of your upper torso will follow. As you

do this, reach around the chair where the bolster is positioned and bear-hug the upright bolster on the chair seat with your left arm to steady yourself. Place your noggin on the portion of the bolster that's above the chair back. Now you're ready to reap the maximum benefits of this pose.

Try to "open" your chest up. With your head on the bolster and a straight back,

JERRY SAYS

"Make sure you have good heel-arch alignment. Nice! Somewhere Fred Astaire is very happy."

place your free arm behind your back. Chest more open? Good. This is where Jerry talks about his shoulder "eye" looking up at the ceiling. Remember, yoga metaphor. I've never seen him with his shirt off, but I bet he doesn't have an eye there.

For a greater opening of the chest, raise your arm toward the ceiling. I always like to point to show who's number one in the class, but that's optional. Try to keep your front leg as straight as possible—that's mandatory. "Remember to breathe," Jerry will tell us. It's not like you're underwater. You merely want to maintain that slow, steady yoga breath during the pose and keep a straight front leg. Just like the three sides of a triangle, this pose has three facets to consider while doing it: straight front leg, head on bolster, arm pointed up to show who's number one.

To come out of this pose, reach for the sky with your free hand and—using your belly muscles—pull yourself upright.

Now move the chair to the opposite end of the mat and the bolster to the opposite side of the chair. Reverse your stance and make like a triangle on your other side with your back against the imaginary wall, nice heel-arch alignment, right thigh setting in hip socket, left arm behind your back or in the air. Breathe and come back out by using your core.

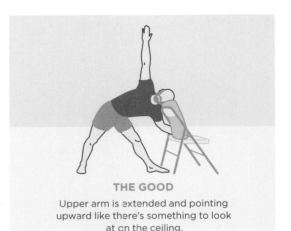

THE GOOD
Upper arm is extended and pointing upward like there's something to look at on the ceiling.

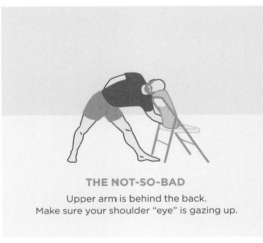

THE NOT-SO-BAD
Upper arm is behind the back. Make sure your shoulder "eye" is gazing up.

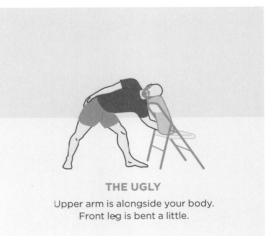

THE UGLY
Upper arm is alongside your body. Front leg is bent a little.

Revolved Triangle Pose
(*Parivrtta Trikonasana*) with Chair and Bolster

Don't lose that chair or bolster yet. You're not done playing the triangle. This is like triangle pose with chair and bolster, the sequel. The pose is called *parivrtta trikonasana*, which is actually really fun to pronounce. Try it yourself. Even better, the movement incorporates a gentle spine stretch.

With your chair at the right side of the mat and the bolster upright on the right side of the chair, place your right foot forward. Step back with your left foot. Unlike the previous triangle pose, your rear foot is positioned a bit wider, which rotates your left hip forward more. That's one of the differences here. The other one is your *left* hand comes around the bolster when you bend sideways at the waist, revolving your torso. It adds a little torque to it. Lean forward and your head should be resting on the bolster again. Open up the shoulder "eye."

For most, this might be more challenging than the previous pose, from a balance perspective. You may just want to keep the right arm along your side instead of reaching for the ceiling. Your call. Breathe calmly.

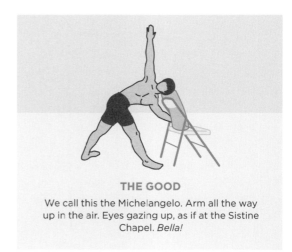

THE GOOD

We call this the Michelangelo. Arm all the way up in the air. Eyes gazing up, as if at the Sistine Chapel. *Bella!*

To come out of this asana, bring your right hand back to the chair and use your core to raise yourself to your full evolutionary height. Move the chair to the opposite end of the mat and place the bolster on the other side of the chair. With your left leg forward, step back with the right, placing your foot wide so that your hips are more rotated. Lean forward, reaching with the right hand around the bolster. Just like before, rest the melon on the cushion and open up the shoulder "eye." Bring the arm around your back or stretch it up toward the ceiling. Breathe. Place your left hand back on the chair and stand up.

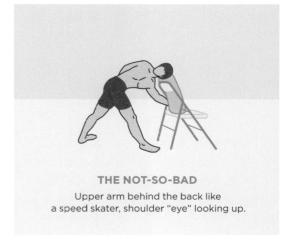

THE NOT-SO-BAD

Upper arm behind the back like a speed skater, shoulder "eye" looking up.

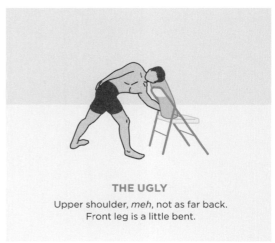

THE UGLY

Upper shoulder, *meh*, not as far back. Front leg is a little bent.

Extended Side Stretch
(*Utthita Parsvakonasana*) with Chair and Bolster

You're already in position for this next one, *utthita parsvakonasana*. Leave your bolster where it is on the chair. This pose is such an extended side stretch, it relieves stiffness in the shoulders and back and gives you a good hamstring/groin stretch. Wow! That's a lot of body parts.

Start with the chair to your left, the back of the chair facing you, and bend your left knee without letting the knee go past the ankle. A good way to gauge that is to always make sure you can see your big toe.

Extend your right leg out straight behind you, front heel aligned with the back foot's arch. Slide your upper torso down using your waist as a hinge, and grasp the base of the bolster with your left arm. If your head isn't resting on the bolster, extend your right leg back until it does. Good, this takes your neck out of the equation.

Jerry hasn't forgotten about your right arm. This is where you're going to reach with a straight arm along the contour of your head, stretching the entire right side of your body, from fingertips to the sole of your foot. It should roughly look like you're pointing at something as you hide behind a wall (the chair back). Reach and breathe.

JERRY SAYS

"Yoga should always be calm and pleasurable. Find your limit and see if it changes as you gain experience."

Then breathe and reach. You're good at this. You must have done this before.

Push the outer rim of your back foot into the floor. The palm of your left hand should be facing the floor. Check to make sure your arm is over your head, not in front of you. If need be, imagine there's a wall behind you. It'll keep you in perfect alignment. Work on straightening that right arm.

To emerge from this pose, straighten the front leg. Just like that, you're back in triangle pose. Then pull yourself up, relying on your core.

Repeat on your other side, with your right leg forward, knee over the ankle, but not obscuring the big toe. Then your torso slides back down the imaginary wall, while extending the left leg straight back until your head is supported on the bolster (right arm hugging the bolster at its base). Reach and point. Breathe. Stretch the e-n-t-i-r-e length of your left side. Do you hear that? It's your groin, shoulders, and back relaxing. Now straighten your front leg to come out of this *asana* into triangle pose and use your core to pull yourself back into a standing position.

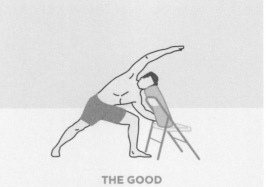

THE GOOD
Your is arm stretched straight over your head.

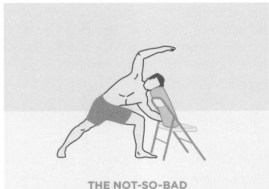

THE NOT-SO-BAD
A less oblique angle. Your elbow might be bent.

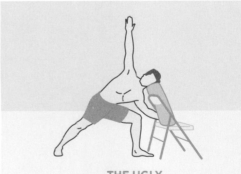

THE UGLY
Even less arm stretch. Less extension to your top shoulder. Maybe you have an actual wall at your back—aka the Yoga Matt way.

Half-Moon Pose (*Ardha Chandrasana*) with Chair and Bolster

This is the last of the vigorous poses in this series of *asanas*. Besides stretching your hamstrings, *ardha chandrasana* improves your balance and strengthens your core. You're already set up to do it because we're going to keep the chair right where it is with the bolster upright on the left side of your chair.

Ready to go whole hog on the half-moon pose? Okay. Step away from the chair 12 to 18 inches, depending on your height. Keep your left leg there and then step back with your right foot roughly 18 inches, establishing a nice heel-arch alignment between the two feet.

I'm not going to lie to you: this one's sort of a toughie. But I know you're man enough to do it. Bend the front knee enough for you to lean forward and grab the base of the bolster while resting your head on the top. You might need to recalibrate your distance from the chair and bolster so that your head rests on the bolster comfortably.

Here comes the tricky balance part: straighten your front leg and lift your back leg up so it's parallel to the ground. Last, your right arm comes up and reaches toward the ceiling, and you look up at your right hand if you can. Even though it looks like you're being pulled in two different directions, your breath should be calm.

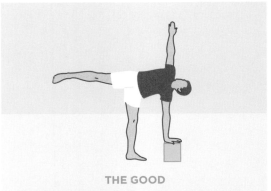

THE GOOD

No chair. No bolster. No problem. (Well, maybe use a yoga block instead of a chair for stability.)

To emerge from *ardha chandrasana*, bend your front leg a bit, and then bring your rear leg back to the floor and straighten your front leg, placing you in triangle pose. From here, use your core to pull yourself upright. You still have the other side of your body to half-moon. Move the chair to the opposite end of the mat. Right leg forward, step back with the left. Hey, keep that head atop the bolster. How's that heel-arch alignment? With a slight bend to the front knee, lift your left leg up horizontal to the floor. Left arm goes up toward the ceiling. Hold for four or five yoga breaths.

Finish by stepping back into triangle pose and, relying on your core, pull yourself up into an upright position. Jerry likes to promise that someday we'll all be doing *ardha chandrasana* without the chair and bolster. Can't wait. I think maybe he's kidding us. It's been about a year of classes and nobody's there yet.

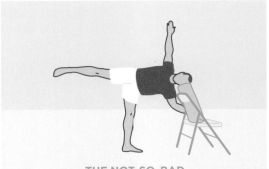

THE NOT-SO-BAD

Perform the pose with a chair and bolster. Maintain a horizontal leg and arm perpendicular to it, pointing straight up.

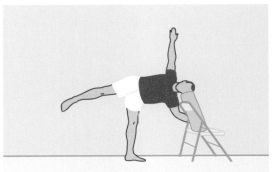

THE UGLY

Position yourself next to a wall for stability and use that chair and bolster. Straight leg as horizontal as you can comfortably maintain.

Downward Dog (*Adho Mukha Svanasana*) and Child's Pose (*Balasana*)

You've already done one version of downward dog. Frankly, there are a lot of ways to do the dog, which gives you lots of flexibility in how you stretch your hamstrings and shoulders, two key areas where guys store stress.

This downward dog is a bit more advanced than the one in the Manly Yoga Practice No. 1. You don't need the chair. Start on your mat on all fours, hands positioned under your shoulders, hips and knees at right angles. Tuck your toes. (Pull your heels off the floor, which places your weight on your flexed toes.) Press into your hands and start straightening your legs so you form an upside-down V.

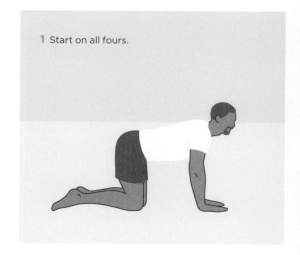

1 Start on all fours.

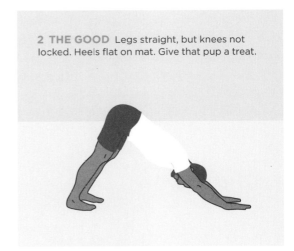

2 THE GOOD Legs straight, but knees not locked. Heels flat on mat. Give that pup a treat.

Sometimes Jerry tells us to imagine our hands are outwardly unscrewing the top of a jar. Really, it's just a way to remove wrist strain from the equation. Let the stretch go wide between your shoulders and let your head hang loose. Can you lift your kneecaps up? This is more of a muscular motion, which engages the quads and helps strengthen your core and align your pelvis. Next, drop your heels. A bit harder than with the chair, isn't it?

Breathe in and out for a few rounds. Then bend your knees and come back down onto all fours, knees on the mat.

CONTINUED

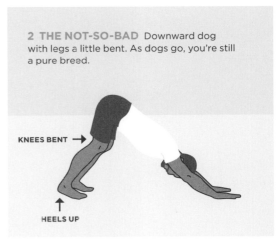

2 THE NOT-SO-BAD Downward dog with legs a little bent. As dogs go, you're still a pure breed.

KNEES BENT →

↑
HEELS UP

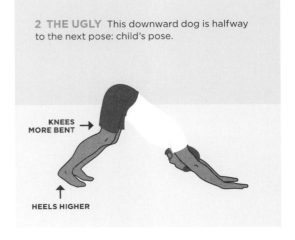

2 THE UGLY This downward dog is halfway to the next pose: child's pose.

KNEES
MORE BENT →

↑
HEELS HIGHER

Downward Dog (*Adho Mukha Svanasana*) and Child's Pose (*Balasana*)

CONTINUED

From here, you'll transition into child's pose. Spread your knees wide, sit back on your heels, and untuck your toes. Your torso leans forward like you're bowing down in submission (or, I suppose, like a crawling infant). Arms can be extended forward in front of you, palms down on the floor. As an alternative, you can bring your arms back along your sides with your hands down by your feet, palms up. Do whatever feels right to you. Child's pose offers a brief form of constructive rest before you get all canine again. Breathe and contemplate that last sentence.

JERRY SAYS

"No matter which variation of downward dog you choose, try to take your wrists out of the equation. Spread your fingers out to equally distribute your weight, hands with a slight outer rotation."

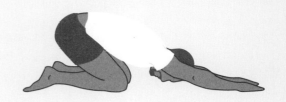

3 Here, child's pose, a form of constructive rest. You're welcome.

Bring yourself up into down dog one more time. Remember to tuck your toes, then straighten your legs and come up. Spread the stretch across your shoulders. Head should be hanging loose, hang-dog style. Lift the kneecaps, drop the heels, breathe.

Come back down to all fours and untuck your toes. Return to child's pose, bent over your legs like a rug rat learning to crawl. Last, roll up into a seated position for the next *asana*.

Seated Forward Bend
(Paschimottanasana)

Great news! You can do this next pose sitting down. The *asana* is called *paschimottanasana*. (A spelling bee in Sanskrit must be hell.)

Once more, this is for the hamstrings and lower back. Guys can't stretch those areas of the body enough. Think of a tightly strung violin. That's us in the hammies and lower lumbar region.

To do *paschimottanasana*, all you need is a mat, a chair, and a blanket. Orient your mat perpendicular to the wall and place the chair against the wall on top of the mat (back facing the wall, seat facing you). Deposit the blanket on the chair seat.

Now sit on your mat facing the chair, legs extending under the seat, knees straight. Wiggle around a little so your bones feel like they're supporting you like railroad tracks. Lean forward toward the chair while keeping your legs flat on the floor. Rest your head on your blanket to relieve neck strain. Let your arms fall like limp macaroni at your sides. Are you breathing? Of course you are. But it shouldn't be like you just finished the Boston Marathon. Easy does it.

THE GOOD

Head on chair, decent forward bend,
legs straight under chair.

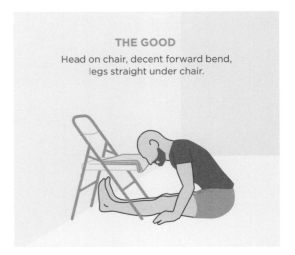

You'll know whether this position is too extreme if you need to bend your knees.
No bad: Simply turn the chair around so the back is facing you. Place the blanket over the chair back and rest your head on the blanket for a more relaxed angle, making it easier to straighten the legs. Arms should still be noodles. Breathe into the stretch.

The overall purpose here is to get the pelvis and legs straight at the same time.
If you have to, modify the position of your chair and blanket to achieve that anatomical arrangement. That's it.

THE NOT-SO-BAD

Head on chair back, body more upright,
legs straight.

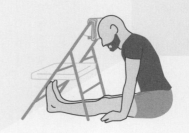

THE UGLY

Even less of a forward bend. If you have to bend your knees a bit, fine. Breathe into your tightness. Ugliness is only a state of mind.

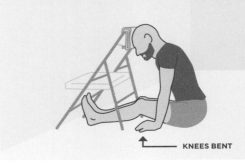

KNEES BENT

Legs Up the Wall

If life has you climbing the walls, there's nothing quite like legs up the wall. It's like a chill pill for stress relief minus the pharmaceutical. Better for you, in other words. Let's keep Big Pharma out of the yoga equation. Tough day at work? Grab a wall instead of a pill.

Besides relieving stress, legs up the wall relaxes the hamstrings and groin. To get into this pose, sit on a folded blanket with your right hip and shoulder against the wall. Hold the blanket with your left hand to ensure the blanket doesn't slide. Then imagine you're a washing machine and rotate a half cycle around so that your head and torso are flat on the floor with your legs miraculously reaching straight up the wall (see diagram). Make sure your sacrum, the triangular bone at the bottom of your spine, is on the floor. Keep your legs straight and engage your leg muscles.

JERRY SAYS

"Whenever you get out of an inversion, take your time. Your heart's been level with or over your head. Stay down on the mat for a few breaths. It's a blood pressure thing."

"This is not a sleeping pose," Jerry frequently explains. "Your legs should be engaged." He doesn't mean they're getting married. It's about achieving a moderate stretch. Breathe your yogiest of yoga breaths. Nice and slow. Can't you just feel that stress dripping away? For maximum relief, 4 minutes is the minimum amount of time to perform legs up the wall. It gets better and better the more you do it. Fifteen minutes before bed is absolutely sublime.

While still in this pose, take your legs wide. You just did *supta upavistha kona-sana*, or reclined wide angle pose. I think of it as the wishbone. Whatever you call it, hold the pose for a few breaths.

Last, stay on your back and bring your legs back together. Bend both legs so that the soles of your feet are touching against the wall, bent knees pointing in opposite directions, thighs pressed against the wall. Move the feet down the wall toward your pelvis. Your bent legs should resemble a butterfly. You can position your hands to press a bit at your hip creases to further open this cobbler, sunnyside up pose.

Breathe. See if that loosens any tightness. If not, breathe deeply and focus on opening up the area.

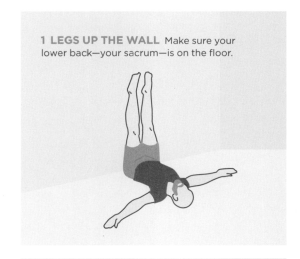

1 LEGS UP THE WALL Make sure your lower back—your sacrum—is on the floor.

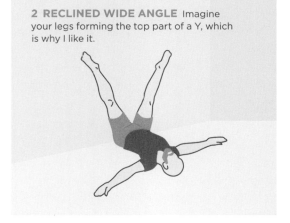

2 RECLINED WIDE ANGLE Imagine your legs forming the top part of a Y, which is why I like it.

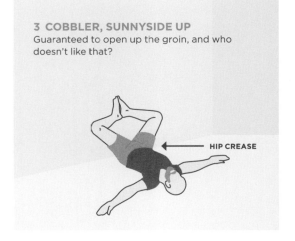

3 COBBLER, SUNNYSIDE UP Guaranteed to open up the groin, and who doesn't like that?

HIP CREASE

Seated Twist

Upper bodies. Men have them and often our upper bodies are stiff or sore from all the manly tasks we're asked to do. Like sitting in a car in traffic. It can be murder on the hips, lower and upper back, and neck.

This seated twist is your antidote. First off, you need something to sit on—a bolster or a couple of blankets. It's kind of like you're shimming yourself up until your pelvis is aligned straight up and down, not tilted back, which is a natural tendency for human beings.

Sit with your legs out in front of you. Orient your feet so the outsides are parallel. None of that splayed Charlie Chaplin feet. Take your right foot over your left thigh and see if you can place the foot on the ground; the closer it's planted to the knee, the better. Go ahead, I'll wait for you.

Then reach your left arm behind your back, with your palm lying flat or up on your fingertips or knuckles—whatever gives you a solid perch as you begin the twist. Remember that right leg that you placed over your left thigh? Your right arm goes outside the raised knee, with the elbow bent and the forearm poised straight up and down, if you can, or out level. Inhale to open your chest. Exhale and twist to the left a little more. Hold it for three calm yoga breaths.

Next we'll twist to the other side. Don't unwind yourself yet. Keep your legs exactly as they are positioned, but switch arms. Your right hand is placed behind you to steady you like the third leg of a tripod. Your left hand is placed on the outside of your raised knee. See the illustrations, especially if you have trouble telling left from right like Yoga Matt does. This one's a little tougher, isn't it? Stop complaining. Give me three long yoga breaths.

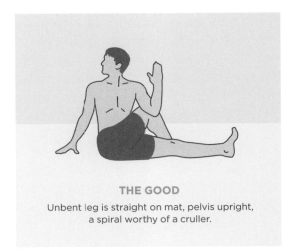

THE GOOD

Unbent leg is straight on mat, pelvis upright,
a spiral worthy of a cruller.

**Unwind, but don't take that victory lap
quite yet.** You still have the other side.
For those of you who forgot the dance
steps: left foot over right thigh. Right arm
reaching back, left arm on the outer side
of your right, bent knee. Inhale and open
your chest, exhale and twist three times,
each time progressively further or as far
as you're comfortable going. Reverse
your arms—left hand behind you, right
arm up and over your knee. Three yoga
breaths. Unwind.

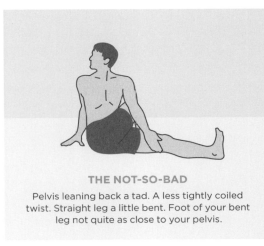

THE NOT-SO-BAD

Pelvis leaning back a tad. A less tightly coiled
twist. Straight leg a little bent. Foot of your bent
leg not quite as close to your pelvis.

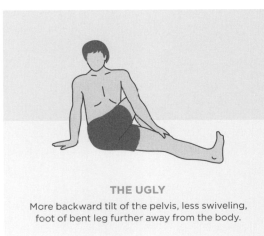

THE UGLY

More backward tilt of the pelvis, less swiveling,
foot of bent leg further away from the body.

Resting Pose, the Sequel (*Savasana*)

Just like there are many ways to perform downward dog, *savasana* isn't a one-trick pony either. It's good to vary the pose so you don't get into a rut. We're talking about your peace of mind. Think of *savasana* as a river of many streams that all flow into the same place, which is known as the Land of Calm.

***Savasana* is just as important as any other *asana* in this book, a chance to stay in the practice for a few more moments before the world comes crashing back.** Unlike other poses that involve the body more directly, *savasana* might be the toughest because it involves keeping the mind engaged. You can reflect on the practice you just performed.

Or best yet, simply focus on your breath for the purest *savasana* experience. One way is following the third breath technique: inhale into your pelvis, then your belly, then your upper chest (see page 53). Exhale and let the air float right out of your body without a sound.

Another breathing exercise is to imagine you're inhaling into the front part of your body and then the back. Exhale anyway you wish, unless it involves whistling.

You've already done the legs-up-the-wall variation of *savasana*, which is a stone-cold classic. Another method is to prop a block under a bolster for a nifty slanted-back pose, like you're catching some rays in a deck chair.

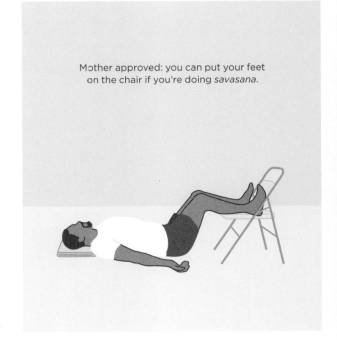

Mother approved: you can put your feet on the chair if you're doing *savasana*.

Or, as we've indicated here, just get a real chair. We've already been using it for the seated twist. Don't put it away just yet. Instead, place your chair at the end of the mat. Jerry likes to pad the seat of the chair with a blanket.

Sit in front of the chair on the mat and lie back. A pillow under the head might be in order, too. Bend your knees and put your feet up on the chair. Position yourself so that your hips and knees are at right angles.

Breathe. If you begin to cogitate about all the things you have to do after this final pose, you're not doing *savasana* right. It's your time to take nothingness seriously. Space out. Enjoy. It's impossible to pronounce *savasana* without a smile. See for yourself.

MANLY YOGA PRACTICE NO. 3

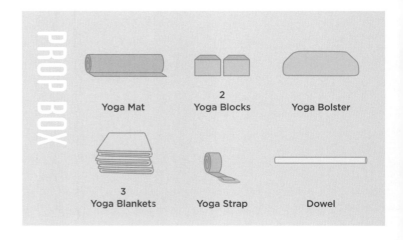

PROP BOX

Yoga Mat

2
Yoga Blocks

Yoga Bolster

3
Yoga Blankets

Yoga Strap

Dowel

Same drill, but different *asanas*. We'll need an hour of your time. Presumably, you've rested for a couple of days since the last time I saw you. The yoga police don't like it if you overdo it (there's really no such thing as the yoga police; yoga Santa Claus, yes).

Jerry's got you doing legs up the wall right from the start. After the wall, Jerry has a few floor poses. You get to imitate a happy baby. In another, straps are involved, but in a very PG way. Jerry even introduces his foot dowels that are just out of this world. All in all, a Manly Practice that's bursting at the seams.

Sixteen different poses. Maybe even seventeen. Yoga Matt usually loses count. That's because I'm thinking of all the healthful qualities that this third Manly Practice promotes. It truly enhances your outer and inner balance because Jerry's got your kidneys, thyroid, and prostate covered. (Insert puerile organ joke here.)

As for your mind, stress takes wing like a supersonic jet. The yoga *asanas* in this practice—and yoga in general—kill stress right in its tracks. The body's no good unless the mind works in sync with it.

Now I know that Jerry—and me by proxy—has placed you in a lot of awkward positions in this book. The last one I want to leave you in, however, is one of calm. This is where I cue the lonely harmonica and get all philosophical. It's just that yoga does that to me. It's not just a great-sounding name. At the end of the class—and the day—yoga is about the breath.

"Yoga *is* breath," Jerry always advises. It took a while for exactly what that meant to sink in, even for metaphorical ol' Yoga Matt. But I think I finally understand. Breath is life, don't you see? And, unless the transitive law of math hasn't been rescinded, what Jerry's really talking about is that yoga is life. That's the secret. Now practice it two or three times a week for as long as you can.

Legs Up the Wall to Reclining Pigeon Pose
(*Supta Kapotasana*)

Legs up the wall at the beginning of the practice is a fantastic warm-up. Get your legs up the wall the way that works best for you. Make sure your sacrum is supported by the floor. Remember that every practice begins with a focus on relaxed breathing. Panting like a dog is considered bad breath.

Your legs should be engaged. Again, they're not getting married (although they are alongside one another on the wall). It means stretch the leg muscles gently. Place your arms on the floor, palms up and keep some space under your armpits. Now's a good time to start the slow, calm breath. Reach down to each hip crease with a hand and push your thighs away from your hips. Try to get some space in there.

Next, take your legs wide. Hands to hip creases again, pushing thighs away. Bring the soles of your feet together and let your knees go wide like butterfly wings. (They pay Yoga Matt the big bucks for metaphors like that.) Bring those heels down the wall as close to your pelvis as you can. Place your hands at your hip creases and push your thighs toward the wall and breathe.

Push harder on the right side, moving your right knee closer to the wall. Your left knee will come off the wall. Go back to neutral and give your left bent leg the same treatment. Again, your opposite knee will come off the wall. Last, use your hands to pull your knees together so you don't tighten any parts you loosened.

Now time to turn into a pigeon. Put your feet hip-width apart on the wall and push away from the wall until your thigh bones are straight up and down and your shins are parallel to the floor.

Position your right ankle over your left knee. Flex your right foot: it protects your knee. It's fine if this is how comfortable you are turning into a pigeon.

To go further, take your right hand through the "hole in the wall" (the opening your bent shin and thigh form) and reach with both arms to hold your left thigh.

For even more, pull your left thigh in the direction of your chest so that your left foot is off the wall. If you're happy here, stop. To go whole pigeon, you can straighten your left leg, take your hand out from the hole in the wall, and start working both hands up toward your foot. Jerry promises eventually you'll be able to grab your toe. (I think he's pulling your leg.)

Put your foot back on the wall and repeat on the other side. Left ankle over right knee, flex the foot. Game for more? Put your hand through the hole in the wall of your bent legs and place both hands around your thigh. See if you can pull that foot off the wall. If you can do that, consider straightening your leg. Maybe even walk your hands up your leg.

To finish, put your feet back on the wall. Slide your feet down toward the floor and push away with your feet until your legs are straight. Keep your feet against the wall so you're ready for your next pose.

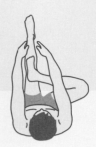

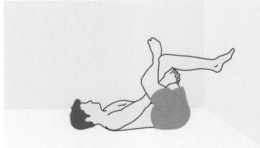

THE GOOD

Pigeon pose, with one leg extended and hands reaching up near your ankle.

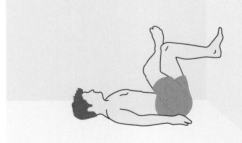

THE NOT-SO-BAD

The species of pigeon where your hands are encasing your thigh and your foot is off the wall.

THE UGLY

Pigeon pose with ankle over one knee, one foot on the wall. All animals are beautiful.

Side Stretch and Floor Twist

Pigeon at the wall flows seamlessly into this next pose, which is side stretch and floor twist. Just the thing for taking the ouch! out of your lower back.

Lie back on your mat with legs straight out flat on the floor, feet in good contact with the wall. Float your arms up toward the ceiling sleepwalker style, right out in front of you at the shoulders. "We're always grabbing at things," Jerry usually admonishes. "This is different. Just let the weight of the arms settle into the shoulder sockets."

Next, bring your arms directly outstretched over your prone head, palms facing each other without touching. Rotate your straight arms back over your head, and keep your hands hovering above the floor a few inches. With your right hand, grab your reaching left wrist. Use your right hand to increase the stretch of your left arm and push into the wall with your left foot. That's it. Get a nice stretch on the entire left side of your body. Breathe in and out and give your other side the same treatment. Left hand grabs the right wrist. Reach with the right arm while you push your right foot into the wall.

We're going diagonal now. Same pose except when your right hand grabs your left wrist again to stretch your left arm, push the right (opposite) foot into the wall. Because yoga appreciates symmetry the way an OCD person does, you have to do the same diagonal stretch in the other direction: left hand to right wrist and stretch the right arm while pushing the left foot into the wall.

We're going to finish up with a twist, the non–Chubby Checker version (if I have to explain that reference to you, you're probably too young for this book). Start by bending your right knee toward the chest, then with your left hand, gently guide your right foot so that it's positioned on the floor on the other side of your left thigh. Swing your right kneecap all the way to the left, down to the floor (it'll bring your right hip up, which is fine). Let your right arm float up into the air. Move it around in the shoulder socket, then after a few yoga breaths take that arm and stretch it flat out on the floor while you keep your knee on the floor. To come out of this stretch, use your core (your abs and inner belly muscles) to pull your right leg back up and reestablish contact with both feet touching the wall, legs out straight.

Second verse, same as the first (except other side). Bend your left knee toward the chest, left foot over right thigh, before taking your left knee all the way to the floor. Your left hip will come up accordingly. Float your left arm above you in the air, moving it around in the shoulder socket. Then your left arm goes out 90 degrees while your knee is still on the ground. Hold the pose for a few breaths and pull yourself back into starting position, reestablishing contact with the wall with both feet.

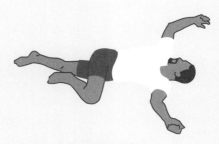

THE GOOD

Finish with a twist. Knee on bent leg is all the way to the floor, pedal to the metal.

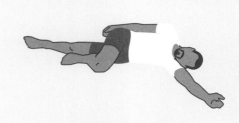

THE NOT-SO-BAD

A more relaxed swivel.
Bent leg is not all the way to the floor.

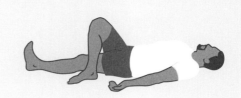

THE UGLY

Hardly any swivel. You're on the ground, foot on the other side of the knee.
Good enough.

Hips and Straps

You're already lying down from the previous pose. Stay there. It keeps your back supported so no one gets hurt. Oh yeah, have a strap handy.

Have both feet in good contact with the wall with your legs straight. Bend your right knee toward your chest and place your hand on the top of your kneecap. The knee is as far as you have to go. Start to slowly rotate your hip in its socket. Nice big circles. Both directions, like a giant clockface and time is moving backward and forward. Breathe and rotate. Now the other direction and breathe.

Next, put the strap over the sole of your right foot. Grasp an end of the strap with each hand and straighten the leg and both arms. Are you breathing that slow, calm breath?

Place both ends of the strap in your right hand and position your left arm straight out to a T. Gaze out over your left hand. Keep that left thigh down, as if it's a horror movie and Jason's nailed it to the floor.

Now take your strapped right leg all the way off to the right, keeping your left thigh and hip nailed to the floor. Breathe and use your core to pull the leg back up to twelve o'clock. Move the strap to the left hand, put your right arm out to a T, and take your right leg to the left, across your body. Keeping both hips on the floor is more important than how far you can take your leg across your body.

Breathe and pull the leg up with your core again, remove the strap from your foot, and bring your foot back to the floor with a bent knee before straightening your leg to reestablish contact with the wall. "Your right leg," Jerry typically notes, "should feel different from the left." He means limp and noodly, in a good way.

It's not yoga if you don't do the other side. Bend the left knee. Hand on that side of the body goes to the kneecap. Rotate your leg in the hip socket. Both directions. Slowly. It's not a race. Big circles.

Grab the strap and place it over the sole of your left foot. Grasp the strap with your right and left hands, arms go water-skier straight. Then, holding both ends of the strap in your left hand, position your right arm off to the right and look over at your right hand.

Breathe and take your left leg wide, down toward the floor on that side. The right leg here should be stapled to the floor. Pull the leg back up to twelve o'clock, relying on your core. Finally, take your left leg to the right, cross-body, while your hips stay on the ground. Your leg will probably get nowhere near the floor, which is fine. You've located your point of resistance—or what's termed your "edge." Congratulations, Columbus, you've discovered the essence of yoga. Breathe. Pull your leg back up to neutral with your core and make contact with the wall with your feet. Your legs should both be as loose as untied shoelaces.

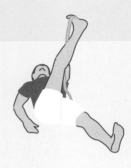

1 12 O'CLOCK HIGH Try to keep a straight leg.

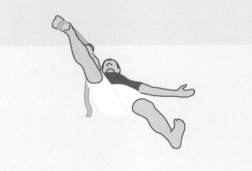

2 WIDE ANGLE Good for the groin!

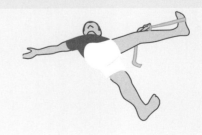

3 CROSS-BODY Keeping both hips on the floor is more important than how far you can cross your leg over your body.

Happy Baby (*Ananda Balasana*)

Who doesn't like a happy baby? In Sanskrit, it's called *ananda balasana*, but no matter how you say it, this pose stretches the groin and spine the best way possible: gently. Happy baby is meant to be a relaxing pose. Anyone with a frown has to do it in the corner of the room facing away. (Just kidding. Jerry's alter ego is a superhero named Captain Inclusive.)

This is considered a warm-up to the more strenuous practice to come. (Cue foreboding soundtrack.) But for now, just start on your sticky mat, lying on the floor on your back, which is pretty much what this third Manly Practice has been majoring in so far.

JERRY SAYS

"You can be any age and still be a happy baby. It's okay, too, if you rock past your tipping point when you tilt!"

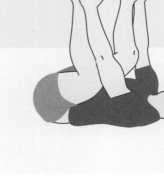

Thighs tight to chest, knees at right angles.
If you're up to it, grab your big toes.
Remember to flex both feet.

Gently bend both knees and bring them up toward your chest. Place your hands on your kneecaps just like in the previous pose and make circles on your sacrum, this time knees together. Tilt to the left to your tipping point without falling over. Then back to neutral, breathing calmly the whole time. Tilt to your tipping point on the right and back to neutral. Travel from one tipping point to the other. If you fall, no problem. Good to know your limits.

Now time for the happy baby part. Bring your knees up high on your chest, each one aimed at the armpit on their respective sides. With the bottoms of your legs, from the knee down, make like you're standing on the ceiling. Your feet should be flexed. With each hand, try to grab a calf apiece. If you can reach up to the outside of your feet, it's known in our class as ecstatic baby.

Next, take your legs wide and hold that for a bit. Breathe and do some wide-legged small circles on your sacrum. A little harder than before, no? Remember, every baby crawls before walking. Try performing the circles in both directions. Come back to neutral, tip left and right. Get to that tipping point and it's fine to tip over. This isn't a DUI checkpoint.

Almost done. Bring your feet back to the floor and gently roll to the right. Face the floor and push yourself up into a seated, cross-legged position on your mat.

Jerry's Salute Pose (*Namaskarasana*)

Lots of classes perform this *asana* at the very beginning. Not Jerry. He's a rebel that way. He thinks it's ideal to do after you've warmed up a little and are properly focused. That Jerry—he gets somewhat philosophical about this pose. "Think about why you're doing yoga," he'll say, "and what you hope to gain."

Wow. I didn't realize that yoga could exercise my brain, too. As you ponder that, sit up on a bolster or your mat. Sit cross-legged, any way you want. Apparently, there are a lot of ways to sit cross-legged in yoga. *Padmasana*, or lotus; *sukhasana*, or regular cross-legged. You choose which leg to fold over the other.

Once you get in a comfortable seated position, reach down and touch the area right under the pad of your big toe on both feet. This should feel great in a totally nonkinky way. Push the toes into

your fingers rather than vice versa. Then repeat with the rest of the little piggies down the line. Don't forget the baby toe. Even the tiniest ones need love.

All of these subtle movements start to engage your base. Don't break that engagement. Bring your elbows out, open your chest, drop your elbows to your sides, and place your hands on your thighs with your palms up, like you're checking if it's raining.

Imagine your thighbones giving in to gravity and dropping. Try to separate your sit bones. It's a muscular shifting, really, that engages your base even more. Then compact your base. Again, one of those muscular things. It's like all the mass in your lower body is anchoring you to the floor. Picture a belt around your knees and around your sacrum, tightening and drawing your base together. Keep all of that. Make sure your head is over your collarbones and your chin is level.

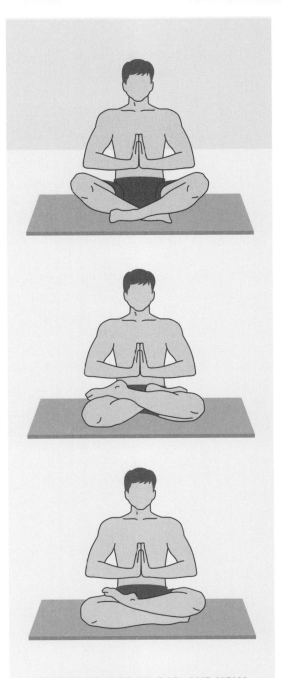

Time to pull your abdominal muscles in toward the spine. Lift the upper part of your body and let your tailbone drop. At the same time, lift the sides of your trunk—not the front ribs—up toward the ceiling while relaxing your shoulders down. The crown of your head reaches for the ceiling. If there's any tightness in the base of your neck, relax it into your throat. Finally, the whole back of your spine softens and moves into the body.

At this point, simply sit, breathe, and quiet your mind. Cooler air in through the nose, slightly warmer air out. Maintain your posture. Bring your hands together at your chest and gently touch the skin of your palms, leaving your fingers splayed. See if you can bring your chin and your chest together by lifting your chest and dropping your chin. A lot of people refer to this as prayer pose. Not Jerry—to him, this is salute pose.

THE GOOD, NOT-SO-BAD, AND UGLY

It's actually all good in *namaskarasana*. Here are three different ways to cross your legs. Always look both ways before you cross.

Wide Wiggly Downward Dog
(Wide Wiggly *Adho Mukha Svanasana*)

This isn't the same old dog. In fact, all three downward dogs in this book are different. The reason it's reprised is that it's a versatile *asana* that covers large muscle groups and can be performed in a number of ways to zero in on specific problem areas within your hamstrings and shoulders.

This species of the dog is as fun as a new puppy, and you're probably already house-trained. *W-dog*, as we sometimes call it, is a slightly more active animal. You start the normal way, on the mat on all fours, but take a wide stance, placing your hands and feet at the edges of your mat. Try to resist the urge to bark. Good dog.

Tuck your toes and press your hands into the mat as you begin to straighten your legs into that upside-down V. Distribute the weight evenly across your hands and fingers; the same across your shoulders.

JERRY SAYS

"Tuck your toes? That's when you're poised on your toes with heels off the ground. Often used in downward dog."

Let your head hang loose. If you can, lift your kneecaps up and drop your heels. But don't pant like a dog. Your breathing should be measured and easy.

Here's the new trick part, a chance to get all wiggly. Bend your knees slowly one at a time, like pistons in slow motion. Stretch your right side and your left. Loosen your shoulders and rotate your head gently from side to side. Put a little rotation in your hips. You're moving about in place, achieving a slow rolling stretch that's designed to enhance range of motion without stressing your body.

Keep doing the wiggly dog for a number of yoga breaths before returning to neutral, bending your knees, and coming down on all fours, hands in front, knees as hind legs. Then bring your hands under your shoulders and your knees hip-width apart. Press your hands into the mat and straighten your legs so that you're back in an inverted V, but this time in the classic downward dog position.

Time to squirm like a puppy again. Legs, hips, shoulders. Everybody does it slightly different in class. If you roughly resemble a dog shaking its pockets to see where it left the car keys, you're doing the pose correctly.

1 THE OLD DOG Hands pressed into the mat. Straight legs. Head hanging low. An even stretch across the shoulders and legs.

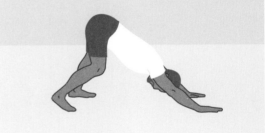

2 WIGGLY DOG, GERMAN POINTER VERSION Bend the knees, one at a time, using your weight to achieve a gentle yet thorough stretch throughout the hamstrings.

3 WIGGLY DOG, NO-FLEAS-ON-ME VERSION Stretch each side out one side at a time. Very slowly like a chewy toy being pulled by two separate dogs. *Rowf!*

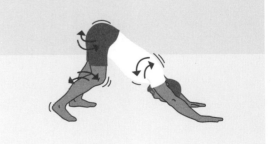

Jerry's Midpractice Foot Massage

This is a Jerry special. I haven't found it in any other yoga book. I think he made it up. The guy's the yoga version of Einstein.

Up until this point, Manly Yoga Practice No. 3 has largely involved *asanas* **where you're down on the mat like a clam.** Or you're on all fours like a dog. For the next poses, it's time to evolve into a biped. Kind of a yoga version of Darwin.

But before you do, Jerry has this neat little way to wake up your feet, a mid-practice palate cleanser, preparing yourself for the standing poses to come. As much as yoga is about physical well-being, it's also about awareness and reengaging with the parts of your body that you take for granted.

Such as your feet. They literally carry the weight of your corporeal world, and how much do you actually think about them? Yoga Matt doesn't want to get all preachy on you, but sometimes he can't help himself.

It's always a treat in class when Jerry pulls out his little bag of dowels. He goes around the room and hands one to each student like a diploma. The idea is to stand and roll the dowel under the sole of one foot on the mat. Focus on the soft area between the foot pads and the heel. "Find the juicy spots," Jerry tells us. "Put as much weight on the dowel as you're comfortable with."

This is the part of the class when a lot of male groaning goes on. Rolling your sole on the dowel hurts so good. There's plenty of nerve endings down there, and you're ironing out the kinks. Work on the inside of the sole, then the outside, and down the middle again.

Step away from the dowel. "If that foot doesn't feel different from the other, you haven't done it right," Jerry says. He means all loosey-goosey and stretched out and *worked*, as if you've had a five-star massage by someone named Gunther.

Your other foot is begging for some of that loving, so repeat on that side. Cue the male groaning. Once the Missus, Beth Matt, heard the class doing Jerry's mid-practice foot massage. (Yoga Matt tapes each session for maximum verisimilitude.) "That doesn't sound like you're doing yoga," Beth said about the chorus of moaning. She has no idea.

This last part is important: pick up the dowel immediately after finishing. Otherwise, it's an accident waiting to happen, an inevitable slip-on-the-banana-peel situation. Don't say you haven't been warned.

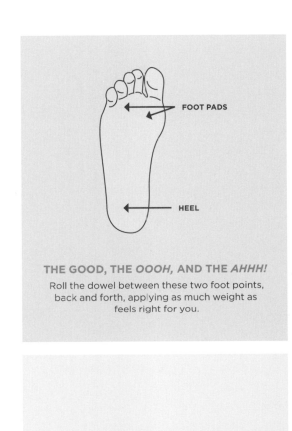

THE GOOD, THE *OOOH,* AND THE *AHHH!*
Roll the dowel between these two foot points, back and forth, applying as much weight as feels right for you.

GET ON THE STICK
A hardware store dowel, 1 inch in diameter, cut into 10-inch sections. Do not proceed to the next asana without putting the dowel away. Remember, this is yoga, a noncontact activity.

Mountain to Eagle Pose
(*Tadasana* to *Garudasana*)

In this one, we're moving from *tadasana* **to** *garudasana***, all without having to go through New Jersey.** Begin in mountain pose, which you've done already. *Tadasana*'s a great starting point for many standing *asanas*.

Stand near a wall with your arms at your sides in mountain pose. (The wall part you might need for balance later.) You're standing with your big toes together or slightly apart, heels separated so the outsides of your feet are parallel. Go ahead, open up your chest. As you stand there, try to lift your kneecaps, which engages the thighs. Arms at your sides, palms facing forward. The crown of your head reaches to the ceiling, but your shoulders drop.

Now step one foot in front of the other and find your balance. Try closing your eyes. Then open your eyes, step back, and reverse your feet so the other foot is forward. Close your eyes again. Open your eyes and go back into mountain pose.

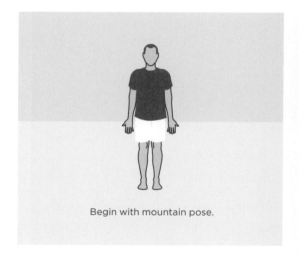

Begin with mountain pose.

Now for the eagle. Put your right leg up over your left as you bend your left knee. (Read that sentence twice; it's got a pretzel logic to it.) Then position your right leg further over your left leg, in order for you to hook your right toe behind your left calf—I kid you not. (See illustration.)

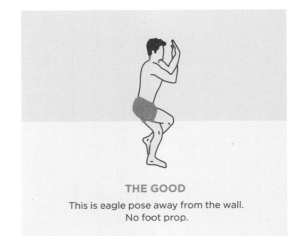

THE GOOD

This is eagle pose away from the wall.
No foot prop.

We're not done. An eagle's got wings. With your right leg over your left already, put your left arm over your right. Continue the twist in your arms to bring your palms around to face one another. Raise your elbows so your upper arms are horizontal to the floor.

That's the ideal. To get there, you might want to start with your back against the wall, to prevent falling over. Alternatively, you can practice on your back on the floor like a fish out of water. In time, when you've acquired a sense of avian balance, you can move away from the wall, squatting low enough so that the foot of the wrapped leg touches the floor, acting like a little kickstand.

Whichever flavor you choose, unwind and do it on the other side. It takes practice to do this one. The full expression of this pose is tough! Start with the simpler versions, from the floor and then the wall. In this one, you have to earn your wings.

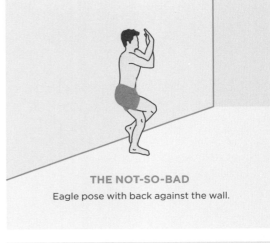

THE NOT-SO-BAD

Eagle pose with back against the wall.

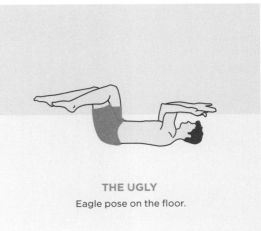

THE UGLY

Eagle pose on the floor.

Warrior 3 (*Virabhadrasana 3*) with Foot on the Wall and Two Blocks

Warrior 3 is excellent for balancing. Jerry uses the wall for this one because, the truth is, men aren't always so great in the balance department.

Even with the wall, this counts as a challenge. It requires core strength. "Maybe someday you'll do it without the wall," Jerry promises. He also says this pose is good for memory and concentration—that part I believe.

Have a couple of blocks handy and position your mat perpendicular to and flush against the wall. Stand about a leg's length away from the wall, facing outward. Orient the blocks vertically, in front of your feet, one on each side, shoulder-width apart. Put one hand on each block for support, then take one leg back so the sole of your foot is flat on the wall behind you. The leg you're standing on should be straight up and down, the other is 90 degrees horizontal and parallel to the floor, and both hands are on the blocks.

Adjust the blocks and your position accordingly to get that right angle with the legs. Now that you're properly aligned, place both feet together on the floor on your mat, and bend over so that each hand is on each corresponding block. Inhale and look up straight ahead. On the exhale, move your right foot back on the wall so your legs are at a right angle. The toes of your raised leg should point toward the floor. If you have sufficient balance, reach your opposite arm out in front of you. Bring your leg back down to the floor. Fold yourself forward like a jackknife for a few breaths of well-earned constructive rest.

Next, with your feet together, do the other side. Inhale and look up. On the exhale, move your left foot back on the wall. Reach with your right arm in front of you, if you're able. Hold it for a few yoga breaths. Then bring your hands back to the blocks and your feet together on the floor.

For the second round of warrior 3, Jerry offers more options than a brand-new car. From your forward fold, inhale, look up, and take your right foot back to the wall. Then take your pick. You can reach your left arm out in front of you. Or bring both arms out to your sides, airplane style. Or, for the thoughtful man, place your palms together and hands to chest, like you're contemplating the many mysteries of yoga. Most challenging of all, you can thrust both arms out in front of you, Superman style.

Finish with your hands on the blocks to steady you, then your foot comes off the wall and back to the ground next to the other one. Don't forget your other side. Exhale and move the left foot to the wall. What you do next with your arms is up to you: right arm out front, both arms like the wings of a 747, hands together on chest, or arms out in front like Superman. Hold the pose for a few calm breaths before bringing your hands back to the blocks and your leg back to the floor. Inhale and look up, exhale, and bend your torso into forward fold.

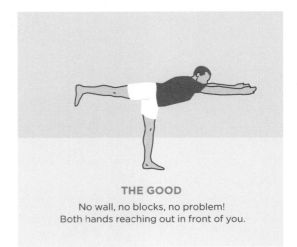

THE GOOD

No wall, no blocks, no problem! Both hands reaching out in front of you.

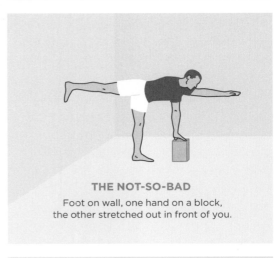

THE NOT-SO-BAD

Foot on wall, one hand on a block, the other stretched out in front of you.

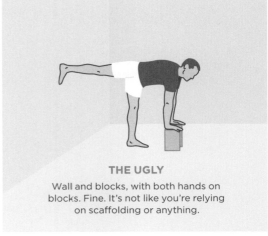

THE UGLY

Wall and blocks, with both hands on blocks. Fine. It's not like you're relying on scaffolding or anything.

Half-Moon Pose (*Ardha Chandrasana*) and Revolved Half-Moon Pose (*Parivrtta Ardha Chandrasana*) with Foot on the Wall

You've already done half of this. The first half. You'll use it to segue into the second *asana*, another example of Vinyasa yoga, which flows from pose to pose. (If you're wondering again, yes, this is all going to be on the test.)

To start, stay where you are from the last pose: standing a leg's length away from the wall. Have that pair of blocks in an upright position in front of your feet, one on each side, shoulder-width apart. Perform a forward fold with your hands on the blocks. Inhale and look up. "Try for a flat back," Jerry says. "No Hunchbacks of Notre Dame. That's a movie."

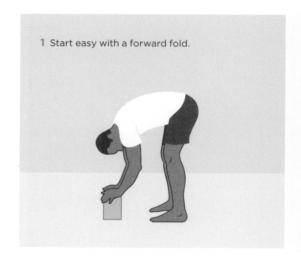

1 Start easy with a forward fold.

2 THE GOOD HALF-MOON The aspirational you: no walls, no blocks. This is how Jerry does it. Show-off.

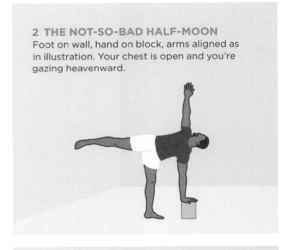

Exhale and bring your right leg to the wall, just like before, at a 90-degree angle—or as close as you can comfortably get to that. Rotate your leg so your toes point toward the side, rather than down toward the floor. Now, to get a little unkinky, let's move that left block over so it's right under your face. (The Sanskrit word for face is *punim*.) Use the block as a support for your left arm. Open up your right arm, stretching your hand up toward the ceiling. If you can, gaze at your raised hand. Breathe. Nice. Right hand goes back to block, with feet together on the floor.

CONTINUED

2 THE NOT-SO-BAD HALF-MOON Foot on wall, hand on block, arms aligned as in illustration. Your chest is open and you're gazing heavenward.

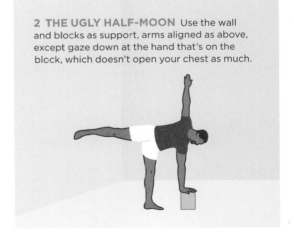

2 THE UGLY HALF-MOON Use the wall and blocks as support, arms aligned as above, except gaze down at the hand that's on the block, which doesn't open your chest as much.

Half-Moon Pose (*Ardha Chandrasana*) and Revolved Half-Moon Pose (*Parivrtta Ardha Chandrasana*) with Foot on the Wall

CONTINUED

Now the other side: inhale, look up, flat back. Exhale and bring your left leg to the wall. Right block is under your face this time and left arm reaches to the sky. Hold the pose for a round of yoga breaths, then return your hand back to the block, take your foot off the wall, and bring your feet together on your mat, hands still on the blocks.

Here's where we evolve into the revolved moon. Inhale, look up. Exhale and take your right foot to the wall. Now, again, we're adding a twist and I don't mean a rhetorical flourish. Place the right block under your face to anchor your right arm and lift your left arm skyward. That's revolved moon (isn't your moon revolved?).

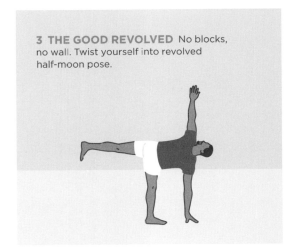

3 THE GOOD REVOLVED No blocks, no wall. Twist yourself into revolved half-moon pose.

Return to earth by bringing your hand back to the block and leg back to the floor in a forward fold. Inhale, look up. Exhale and extend your left foot back flat on the wall. The left block goes under your face to support your left arm and your right arm reaches like you're pointing to a fly on the ceiling directly overhead. Hold, breathe, feel over the moon, then return your raised hand to the block, feet together.

Inhale, look up. Exhale and end with a forward fold, resting for three or four breaths. Last, with slightly bent knees, roll up slowly into a standing position.

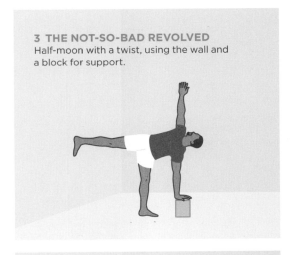

3 THE NOT-SO-BAD REVOLVED Half-moon with a twist, using the wall and a block for support.

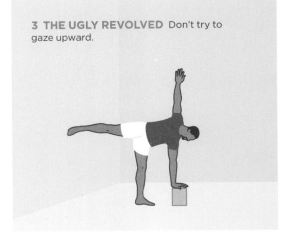

3 THE UGLY REVOLVED Don't try to gaze upward.

Shoulder Stand (*Salamba Sarvangasana*) at the Wall

You'll need three blankets folded into roughly a 1-foot by 3-foot rectangle. Stack one on top of the other. Arrange your mat perpendicular to the wall and place the stack of blankets about a foot from the wall (more if you're taller, less if shorter). Jerry insists the folds must be away from the wall. He must be loads of fun on laundry day.

Take the far end of your sticky mat and fold it over the blankets to hold your shoulders in place when you get into position. I know: it's a lot of directions. But this *asana* is particularly good for fatigue, insomnia, and depression, the big three. So it's worth it. *Salamba sarvangasana* is designed for keeping those hounds at bay.

Orient yourself with your shoulders on the outer edge of your stack of blankets and mat. Then put your feet up on the wall with bent knees.

The least stressful for the shoulders and neck is to keep your sacrum on the blankets, feet on the wall so that your bent knees are at a 90-degree angle. "That's all you have to do," Jerry says.

If you're feeling a bit more rubbery, perform the pose with your shoulders on the sticky mat and the blankets repositioned

JERRY SAYS

"Whatever you do, do not turn your head to the side while you're in shoulder stand. Protect your neck, it's the only thing that holds your head up."

to support your neck and head. Now walk your legs up the wall so you're up on your shoulders. For back support, prop your hands under your sacrum with your elbows on the blankets. It's all good as long as your neck is okay. By that, Yoga Matt means free of pain and stress. Be kind to your neck. Study the illustrations.

Last, if you're doing the second option, try straightening one leg at a time while flexing the foot. If you're fine, try a full shoulder stand, both legs off the wall, toes pointing straight up toward the ceiling.

Hold the *asana* for 30 seconds, then bring your legs down to the mat for some constructive rest. If you still feel like you're climbing the wall, emotionally speaking, one more round is the right medicine. *Salamba sarvangasana* can be habit-forming, but unlike pills, it's not bad for you.

At the end, bring your legs down very slowly. Scoot off the blankets to allow your sacrum to be supported by the mat. Your feet can be up the wall, or you can bend your knees and put your feet on the floor.

The shoulder stand is an inversion, so get up slowly to prevent dizziness. Simply bring your knees to your chest, gently roll to one side, and rest there. Don't just pop up. The change in blood pressure might make you "dingy," according to Jerry.

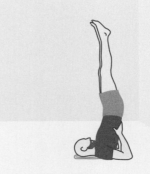

THE GOOD
Away from the wall, both legs up.

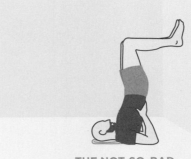

THE NOT-SO-BAD
Feet fairly high on the wall—enough that you're on your shoulders and your back is straight.

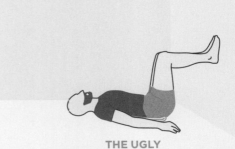

THE UGLY
Feet not so far up the wall. Sacrum on stack o' blankets. You're still reaping the benefits of a solid shoulder and neck stretch.

Boat Pose (*Navasana*) with Strap

Here's one more inversion, which is where your legs are level with or higher than your heart—good for fatigue, insomnia, and depression.

Have a yoga strap handy. Start by orienting your mat so it's perpendicular to the wall. With the yoga strap, make a nice big loop, like you're trying to encircle a giant sequoia.

Lie down on your back. Place the strap around your head, above your ears. Put the soles of your feet inside the other side of the loop and straighten your legs, which will bring your back up off the floor. Play with the neck traction that's most comfortable. Move your legs accordingly. Or reposition the strap—Yoga Matt's tater is so big, it takes some adjusting.

Then move the strap to the back of your neck and find your balance. This is supported boat pose. Just don't overdo it. The idea is to find your balance, like a buoyant vessel. Once you do, stretch your arms out in front of you, pointing to your feet. Ahoy, matey! Remember to breath calmly. Don't make like it's your first tour on the wavy main.

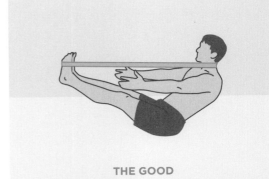

THE GOOD

Legs out straight, arms stretched out in front of you. Body in a nice V shape. Looking pretty good, sailor!

To finish, bend your knees and lie back down. If you're up to it, take the boat out for a few more spins, breathing that long, steady breath. Your call. Whatever floats your boat, so to speak. As with any inversion, take a few breaths, to even out your blood pressure, before righting yourself.

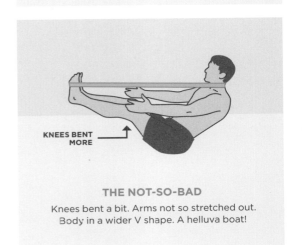

KNEES BENT
MORE

THE NOT-SO-BAD

Knees bent a bit. Arms not so stretched out. Body in a wider V shape. A helluva boat!

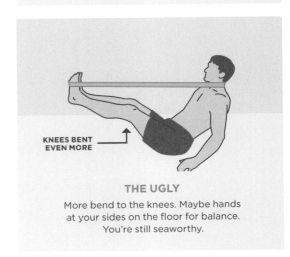

KNEES BENT
EVEN MORE

THE UGLY

More bend to the knees. Maybe hands at your sides on the floor for balance. You're still seaworthy.

Windshield Wipers to Jerry's Favorite Resting Pose (*Savasana*)

Savasana—perhaps the sweetest four syllables of Sanskrit. But before we get to that, Jerry likes to clean the windows. Just some mild windshield wipering with the legs to loosen yourself up for real relaxation. Lie down on your back with your knees bent and feet wide on the mat.

Let your knees slowly flop to the right, left knee toward the right ankle. Stretch your left arm out on the floor, perpendicular to your body, while elongating the rest of that side of the body. Knees come back up and you repeat with your right knee dropping down slowly to your left ankle, while your right arm reaches out to the right, stretching your entire right side. Go back and forth slowly. Bring your knees back to neutral; it's *savasana* time.

Jerry's favorite *savasana* is placing a blankie under his head right up to his shoulders. He also likes a bolster under his knees. Lie back; Charlie Chaplin feet are perfectly acceptable. (If you ever have the time, ask ol' Yoga Matt about his Charlie Chaplin connection.) Palms up with a little space at the armpits.

JERRY SAYS

"Yoga begins and ends with the breath. *Savasana* is a way to reflect on all the yoga goodness you experienced in this practice."

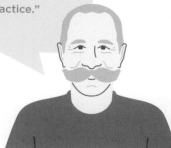

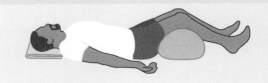

Now, as you reach *savasana* restoration, you have full license to bliss out. Jerry often says, "Yoga is the cessation of the fluctuations of the mind," particularly the practice known as *pratyahara*, which translates into a perfectly legalized way to withdraw from your senses. Relax the skin on the skull. Let it go. See if you can get your eyeballs to rest deep in your sockets. Soften your nose. Let your tongue relax like a limp rope. Imagine your inner ears softening and moving in. They have a Sanskrit word for this that you might not be familiar with: *unplugging*. It's from a strange land where there are no worries.

Your mind—that crazy monkey—might try to start back up. If so, relax the forehead, eyes, nose, tongue, and ears again the way I just showed you.

Yoga Matt's
Final Roll-Up

Well, I guess this is it. Or it's really only the beginning. Kinda Zen, huh? That's the way yoga is, too. It's always surprising you with what it is, a series of poses for the body that also help the mind.

Where to go from here? Start with doing yoga at least two times per week. Don't rush. Each Manly Practice in this book should last about an hour, just like Jerry's class. Always finish up with a few minutes of restorative yoga—legs up the wall or flat-out *savasana*, pick your poison. That old world can spin a bit without you. Vary which series of poses you perform. To finish out the book, you'll find a handy guide for sport-specific muscle groups. All the *asanas* are from this book, we've just reorganized them to cater to specific needs. Once a month, you should undertake a restorative session, which is basically very gentle stretching. "These aren't sleeping poses," Jerry likes to say, but they're pretty close. You can get a PDF of a restorative series by e-mailing restorativeyogamatt@gmail.com.

But the real place all this can take you is yoga without the training wheels. It's already begun to happen in our class. First it was Dave. One week he was there on his mat with the rest of us. The next, he was in the grown-up class with all the yoga regulars. Next it was Orion. Soon it's going to be Quin. In class he has that faraway look in his eyes and can no longer be described as inflexible.

Sometimes the rest of us meet up on the street to watch the two of them in class at Yoga on Center. We press up to the glass outside on the sidewalk. Dave and Orion are totally doing it. They have nothing to be ashamed about. We smile at each other and nod. Someday, we tell ourselves. *Someday . . .*

Sport-Specific Yoga Sequences

If you're a sporty type, yoga can fine-tune that machine you call a body and turn you into a better-performing whole. Unlike the Manly Practices in this book, the series of *asanas* listed on the following pages concentrate on specific muscle groups and body areas used in particular sports.

You'll notice there are only four or five poses. Very perceptive of you. The reason is that you're zeroing in on a narrower group of muscles and you don't ever want to overdo it. Yoga is powerful stuff. A little goes a long way.

We also didn't include a breathing warm-up pose or *savasana*. You're mature enough to pick your favorite at this point. That's not an invitation to skip those segments. Yoga operates on an honor system.

We also didn't include instructions. Instead, we have a handy pictogram and a page number where you can find the pose described in full.

Also feel free to throw mountain pose (page 30) or a forward bend (page 31) into the mix for constructive rest. If you remember to use your breath as your guide, these sport-specific practices should take about 30 minutes, about half the length of our Manly Practices. Perfectly fine. Insert a sport-specific routine once every two weeks into your yoga mix, and you won't believe the kind of good sport you'll turn into.

Running

Legs, hips, and back primarily. Don't forget to breathe. Runners depend on it.

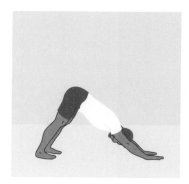

Downward Dog (page 74).
Or if you want a variation on the classic downward dog, try it with a chair (page 28) or try the wiggly version (page 98).

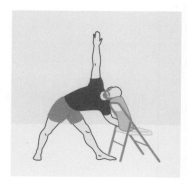

Triangle Pose (page 66)

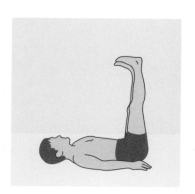

Leg Stretch (page 46)

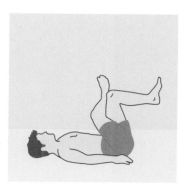

Reclining Pigeon Pose (page 88)

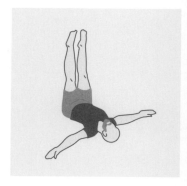

Legs Up the Wall for *savasana* (page 80)

Cycling

Hamstrings, pelvis, and shoulders. Breathing's important in cycling, too. Spinning your wheels and going nowhere is okay if it's *savasana*.

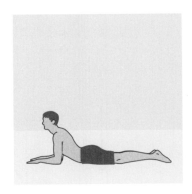

Sphinx (page 58)

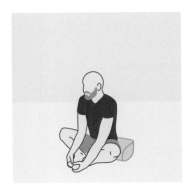

Cobbler's Pose with Forward Bend (page 24)

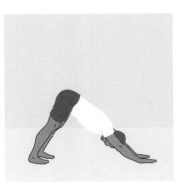

Downward Dog (page 74). Or if you want a variation on the classic downward dog, try it with a chair (page 28) or try the wiggly version (page 98).

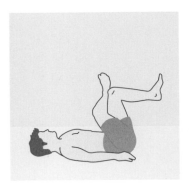

Reclining Pigeon Pose (page 88)

Swimming

Shoulders, arms, back, and legs. We throw you in the deep end. Finish with legs up the wall. More restful than the dead man's float.

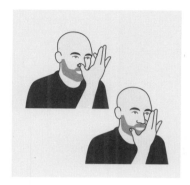

Alternate Nostril Breathing (page 56)

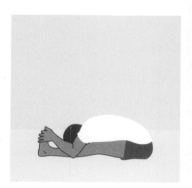

Staff Pose with Forward Bend (page 22)

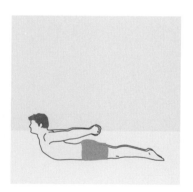

Locust (page 60)

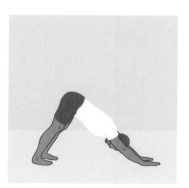

Downward Dog (page 74). Or if you want a variation on the classic downward dog, try it with a chair (page 28) or try the wiggly version (page 98).

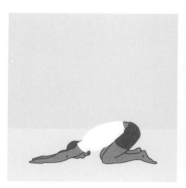

Child's Pose (page 74)

Basketball

Arms, shoulders, neck, and legs. *Asanas* that improve your focus for those shots beyond the arc. Nothing but net!

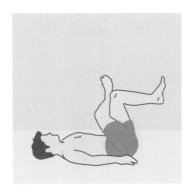

Reclining Pigeon Pose (page 88)

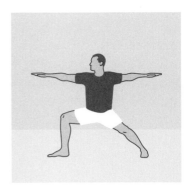

Warrior 2 (page 38)

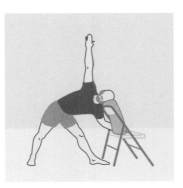

Triangle Pose (page 66)

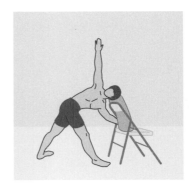

Revolved Triangle Pose (page 68)

Baseball and Softball

Hips, shoulders, and legs. *Soft*ball? There's going to be nothing soft in your game.

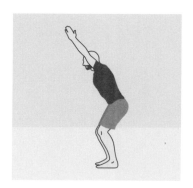

Chair Pose (page 32)

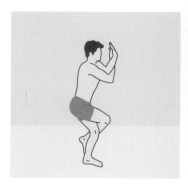

Eagle Pose (page 102)

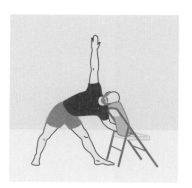

Triangle Pose (page 66)

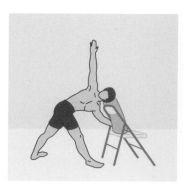

Revolved Triangle Pose (page 68)

Golf

Shoulders, hips, and back.
A focus on stretching all the
long muscles in your body.
Think of it as the secret ingre-
dient of your short game.

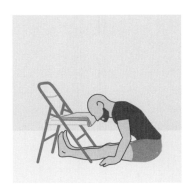

Seated Forward Bend (page 78)

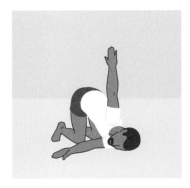

Shoulder Stretch (page 64)

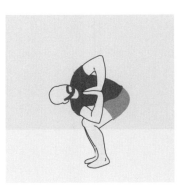

Chair Pose with a Twist (page 32)

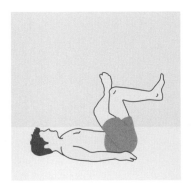

Reclining Pigeon Pose (page 88)

Glossary

This is so you can look like you know what you're talking about if you ever get in a conversation about yoga with someone. Also, it covers a lot of the frequently used terms in the book as well as a few "Jerryisms" that sometimes require further explanation to appreciate their full meaning.

Asana (pronounced AH-sa-na. It took Yoga Matt five months to get this right.) Sanskrit for "yoga pose." If you say it around the yoga studio, you'll sound like a regular.

Charlie Chaplin feet When the toes of your feet are rotated outward. Also called duck feet. Only acceptable in *savasana* when propped on top of a yoga bolster, according to Jerry.

Drishti Focused steady gaze, usually applied at a fixed point that helps anchor you to the floor. A great technique to develop for poses—or *asanas*, for you quick learners—that require balance.

Foot pads The hardened skin under the toes and heels.

Front and back breathing A breathing technique to focus the mind. On the intake, imagine the breath filling the front part of your chest, then the back. Exhale. Repeat. Relax. Breathe.

Heel-arch alignment A stance with the heel of the forward foot pointing straight back, rear foot oriented at a 45-degree angle behind it. An imaginary straight line is formed from the front heel to the arch of the back foot.

Hip crease The hinge your torso forms when seated. Your butt and legs are one plane, upper body the other.

Inversion A term for when you are upside-down or lying down with your feet elevated, as in legs up the wall. Technically it refers to poses when your heart is at a higher level than your head. Downward dog is also a type of inversion.

Iyengar yoga A practice based on this totally hardcore dude, B. K. S. Iyengar, whose idea of yoga pants faintly resembles a diaper and sessions last for hours. Jerry always refers to him as Mr. Iyengar.

Monkey mind When your mind swings around like a caged primate at the zoo, jumping from topic to topic, aka everyday life. The constant barrage of information, interruptions, unfinished thoughts. Everything that yoga offers you a reprieve from.

Namaste A friendly salute to another person, a Hindu version of "nice to see you."

Patanjali The guy who put the OG in Yogi. The first person to assemble the poses into a unified discipline. Another individual Jerry has deep respect for. At the end of class, he asks us to thank Patanjali.

Restorative yoga A slow, gentle practice meant to calm both mind and body. If you practice yoga regularly, it's good to throw in a session of restorative yoga, which involves slow stretches that focus more on the breathing than the stretch. It's like *savasana*'s greatest hits in one simple workout! E-mail restorativeyogamatt@gmail.com to get a PDF. It's Yoga Matt's gift for buying this book.

Sacrum Not a Hindu term. It's anatomical for the triangular bone at the base of your spine.

Savasana The conclusion of every class. Performed a variety of ways: Lying on the floor like a human carpet. Legs up the wall. Legs on a chair. Always combined with breathing techniques, like third breaths, to keep yourself in the moment.

Shoulder eye The hollow under the coat hanger part of your shoulder bone before it reaches the rotator cuff. Jerry's always asking us to point it to the ceiling.

Sit bones The part of your anatomy you feel when you take a seat on an old unpadded football bleacher.

Sun salutation The basis or jumping-off point (metaphorically speaking; it's yoga, not trampolines) for a series of linked poses, intended to honor the big yellow ball in the sky.

Tadasana Mountain pose, the granddaddy of all standing poses. From a yoga perspective, it's as old as the earth. See Yoga Matt's handy mnemonic device (page 30) for mastering this *asana*. It's impossible to forget.

Third breaths A breathing technique to quiet the monkey mind. The intake is divided into thirds. Begin by breathing deep into the pelvis, then higher into the diaphragm, and finally into the upper chest and throat. Then exhale by opening your mouth and letting the breath out without a sound.

Tuck your toes Jerry always says this. Especially during downward dog. It involves positioning your toes like you're in an imaginary sprinter's starting block, toes poised on the ground. Also known as tuck your piggies. (No it's not.)

Vinyasa yoga The coordination of breath with a series of poses that flow from one to another. Jerry's endless sun salutation in Manly Yoga Practice No. 1 is a prime example.

Whirligig See Monkey mind. Jerry calls it the whirligig. I swear, when I'm down on my mat sometimes during *savasana*, he sounds just like Wilford Brimley.

Yoga blanket See "Props," page 10.

Yoga block See "Props," page 10.

Yoga breath Jerry also refers to it as a long, measured breath. Or imagine that a tube runs from the mouth down to the pubic bone. It's a method to ground yourself in the poses as well as calm the busy mind and fidgety body.

Yoga mat See "Props," page 10. When capitalized and spelled with an extra *t*, the author of this book.

Yoga pants Until some fancy company approaches us with a sweetheart deal, we recommend shorts.

Yoga state of mind Calm, measured breathing. Existing in the here and now.

Yoga strap See "Props," page 10.

Yogi Yoga practitioner. That's you after you've read this book. You'll probably need to change your business cards.

JERRY SAYS

"Hey guys, let's do yoga. Three times a week as long as you can."

For the Yoga Curious (Bibliography)

Periodicals

Yoga Journal. Start here. Great, in-depth how-to information on yoga poses. The online version (yogajournal.com) has an extensive yoga pose "library."

Men's Health. Not a ton of yoga but when articles do appear, they are helpful and man-specific.

Books

Brown, Christina. *The Yoga Bible: The Definitive Guide to Yoga.* Hampshire, UK: Godsfield Press, 2003. Over 150 poses, with photos. Something for everyone, beginner to expert.

Brown, Christina. *The Modern Yoga Bible: The Definitive Guide to Yoga Today.* Hampshire, UK: Godsfield Press, 2017. Read on its own or as a companion to *The Yoga Bible* (see above). More-modern poses. Still plenty of photos.

Dederer, Claire. *Poser: My Life in Twenty-Three Yoga Poses.* New York: Farrar, Straus and Giroux, 2010. A memoir about life, marriage, and, of course, yoga. A funny take on yoga from the point of view of the "more-fair" sex.

Iyengar, B. K. S. *Light on Yoga* revised ed. New York: Schocken, 1977. Iyengar yoga, Jerry's specialty. B. K. S. introduced yoga to the West, and there's a whole style of yoga named after him because of it. Go to the source for your yoga poses. Also features an appendix of ailments and the poses that treat them.

Kaminoff, Leslie, and Amy Matthews. *Yoga Anatomy,* 2nd edition. Champaign, IL: Human Kinetics, Inc., 2011. If you're interested in what's going on inside your body during downward dog, this book is for you.

Lacerda, Daniel. *2,100 Asanas: The Complete Yoga Poses.* New York: Black Dog and Leventhal Publishers, 2015. Yup, complete. Every *asana* you could imagine, with a photo of the pose done perfectly.

Matt, Yoga. *More Yoga for the Inflexible Male.**

Mehta, Silva, Mira Mehta, and Shyam Mehta. *Yoga the Iyengar Way.* London: Dorling Kindersley, 1990. With a foreword from B. K. S. Iyengar himself. More than one hundred poses done the Iyengar way, with advice for the beginner and the inflexible. A book after Yoga Matt's heart.

Satchidananda, Sri Swami. *The Yoga Sutras of Patanjali.* Buckingham, VA: Integral Yoga Publications, 2012. Originally published under the title *Integral Yoga: The Yoga Sutras of Patanjali.* Patanjali is Jerry's hero. I swear he must have a poster of him above his bed. Good if you want to delve into yoga's origins.

Singleton, Mark. *Yoga Body: The Origins of Modern Posture Practice.* Oxford, UK: Oxford University Press, 2010. Argues that modern yoga, as practiced by Yoga Matt himself, is derived more from Indian nationalism, bodybuilding, and women's gymnastics than it is from the ancient yoga sutras. Interesting.

Sparrowe, Linda, with *Yoga Journal. Yoga at Home: Inspiration for Creating Your Own Home Practice.* New York: Universe Publishing, 2015. Advice on setting up your at-home practice, with poses and sequences from famous yoga teachers and practitioners. Plenty of photos!

Stanley, Jessamyn. *Every Body Yoga: Let Go of Fear, Get on the Mat, Love Your Body.* New York: Workman Publishing, 2017. Inclusive and informative, with plenty of pose modifications. Ms. Stanley is a *New York Times* yoga expert, so you know there's nothing fake about her.

* A young Yoga Matt can dream, can't he?

About the Author

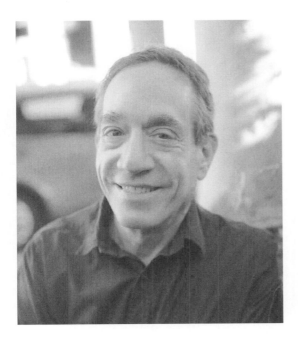

About Yoga Matt

Yoga Matt is the *nom de namaste* of Roy Parvin, an award-winning author of two books of fiction, *The Loneliest Road in America: Short Stories* and *In the Snow Forest: Three Novellas*. He's been the recipient of a National Endowment for the Arts grant in Literature, a Bread Loaf Fellowship, and the Katherine Anne Porter Prize in Fiction. His work has been widely anthologized and included in the Best American Short Stories series. *Voyez Comme Ils Dansent* (director, Claude Miller), a movie adapted from one of Roy's novellas, "Menno's Granddaughter," won the Grand Jury Prize at the Rome 2011 Film Festival. Oddly enough, much like Superman and Clark Kent, Yoga Matt and Roy have never been seen in the same room at the same time.

Yoga Matt's adviser, **Jerry Sinclair**, is an ex-competitive wrestler (the real kind, not that WWF stuff), and has been practicing yoga for more than twenty-three years. He is influenced by the Iyengar tradition of yoga as well as Yogananda and Kali Ray TriYoga. Jerry completed his teacher training course at the Yoga Center of Carmel. His class is a unique blend of supported and meditative *asanas*, *pranayama*, and *pratyahara*. He also takes the award for most flexible man who gets a senior discount.

Acknowledgments

I've often heard it said that it takes a village to raise a child. With *Yoga for the Inflexible Male*, it took a class and the willingness of Jenn Russo and Katina Knapp of Yoga on Center in Healdsburg, California, to take a chance on a guy who never took a yoga class before.

All of my original inflexible classmates—the three Steves, Don, Orion, Quin, Dave, Tod, John, Joe, Thom, Lee, Bruce, Frank, Bill, and that guy in the corner whose name I never caught—have demonstrated rare courage in going where few men have gone before: the yoga studio.

Thanks as well to Patrick Miller of Fearless Literary. I'm lucky to have Kelly Snowden, my wise editor at Ten Speed Press, who laughed when she first heard the idea for this book and then took me very seriously. Isabelle Gioffredi and Betsy Stromberg, who handled the graphics in these pages, are incredible book designers. I've never looked this good on a bookshelf before.

And to Richard Sheppard: fantastic illustrations!

Jerry Sinclair, my yoga instructor, is one of the great teachers I've had in my life. Finally, I have three women to thank for helping birth this very manly book. Monica Kamsvaag created the visual fingerprint for the concept. We'd be nowhere without her. Or Laurie Fox, for that matter, my other agent (Yoga Matt's so important, he has two agents!), who hooked me up with Fearless Literary.

My dear wife, Beth Matt (aka Janet Vail), has been as indispensable to this project as she has been in every other facet of my life. I'm crazy lucky to be married to a publishing professional acquainted with every facet of book production. Beth/Janet has been the invisible spine that binds *Yoga for the Inflexible Male* together. In addition to that, she's laughed at every stupid joke I ever shared with her. To her, I'm funny rather than funny looking.

Index

131

Library of Congress Cataloging-in-Publication Data
Names: Matt, Yoga, 1957- author.
Title: Yoga for the inflexible male : a how-to guide / Yoga Matt.
Description: First edition. | New York : Ten Speed Press, an imprint of
   Random House, [2019] | Includes bibliographical references and index.
Identifiers: LCCN 2019014812| ISBN 9781984856944 (hardcover) | ISBN
   9781984856951 (ebook)
Subjects: LCSH: Yoga. | Exercise for men. | Stretching exercises. |
   Men--Health and hygiene.
Classification: LCC RA781.67 .M38 2019 | DDC 613.7/046--dc23 LC record
available at https://lccn.loc.gov/2019014812

Trade Paperback ISBN: 978-1-9848-5694-4
eBook ISBN: 978-1-9848-5695-1

Printed in China

Cover illustration and design by Isabelle Gioffredi

10 9 8 7 6 5 4 3 2 1

First Edition